Navigating Complexities

Leroy A. Baker

Navigating Complexities

The Intersectionality of Blackness and Disability in Higher Education

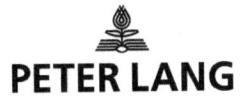

New York · Berlin · Bruxelles · Chennai · Lausanne · Oxford

Library of Congress Cataloging-in-Publication Data

Names: Baker, Leroy A., author.
Title: Navigating complexities : the intersectionality of blackness and disability in higher education / Leroy A. Baker.
Description: New York, NY : Peter Lang, [2025] | Includes bibliographical references and index.
Identifiers: LCCN 2024042360 (print) | LCCN 2024042361 (ebook) | ISBN 9781636677422 (paperback) | ISBN 9781636677439 (pdf) | ISBN 9781636677446 (epub)
Subjects: LCSH: College students, Black—Canada—Social conditions. | College students with disabilities—Services for—Canada. | Educational equalization—Canada. | Racism in education—Canada. | Inclusive education—Canada.
Classification: LCC LC2804 .B35 2025 (print) | LCC LC2804 (ebook) | DDC 371.9/047408996071—dc23/eng/20241018
LC record available at https://lccn.loc.gov/2024042360
LC ebook record available at https://lccn.loc.gov/2024042361
DOI 10.3726/b22394

Bibliographic information published by the Deutsche Nationalbibliothek. The German National Library lists this publication in the German National Bibliography; detailed bibliographic data is available on the Internet at http://dnb.d-nb.de.

Cover design by Peter Lang Group AG

ISBN 9781636677422 (paperback)
ISBN 9781636677439 (ebook)
ISBN 9781636677446 (epub)
DOI 10.3726/b22394

© 2025 Peter Lang Group AG, Lausanne
Published by Peter Lang Publishing Inc., New York, USA
info@peterlang.com - www.peterlang.com

All rights reserved.
All parts of this publication are protected by copyright.
Any utilization outside the strict limits of the copyright law, without the permission of the publisher, is forbidden and liable to prosecution.
This applies in particular to reproductions, translations, microfilming, and storage and processing in electronic retrieval systems.

This publication has been peer reviewed.

Contents

Preface vii
Acknowledgments ix

Introduction 1

Part I Identity: The Visible vs the Invisible
Chapter 1 Blackness 33
Chapter 2 Disability 61
Chapter 3 Intersectionality 85

Part II The Bureaucratic Education System
Chapter 4 Paradoxical Power 111
Chapter 5 Accommodations 163

Part III Confronting and Dismantling
Chapter 6 Embedded Marginalization 221
Chapter 7 Future Directions 233

Appendix A	247
Appendix B	249
Index	251

Preface

I grew up as an abused and neglected youth in Jamaica, and I learned firsthand how these obstacles result in social, economic, and psychological marginalization of the abused male body. After immigrating to Canada, the category of race made my previous challenges more comprehensible. These experiences are part of what motivated me to apply to the Transitional Year Program at the University of Toronto, as an entry to postsecondary education and, later, to pursue an undergraduate degree in Equity Studies.

I enrolled in several courses in disability studies that examined equity and the body; this ultimately encouraged my interest in how individual social position is frequently reflected institutionally. I became interested in critically examining my early challenges living in an abusive family in Jamaica and my experiences immigrating to Canada, and both examinations had several unanticipated benefits. First, these critical examinations served to strengthen my resolve; second, they afforded me a unique opportunity to gain experience occupying marginalized social and material spaces; and finally, they reinforced my belief in the necessary connection between critical thinking and survival, whether that survival is physical, psychological, or intellectual.

The racial, disability, sexual, and gender diversity within my program's student body and my subsequent understanding of the systemic and personal challenges faced by these historically marginalized groups has broadened my understanding of social and educational systems, including their ability to exclude individuals who lack significant power to resist social and institutional exclusion in Canada.

Undoubtedly, my belief in the value and necessity of education comes from my rough personal academic journey over the years; a journey into an unfamiliar environment as a young child who experienced physical violence and social oppression in Jamaica and as an immigrant to Canada who encountered institutional anti-Black racism and personal exclusion. The experiences of Black Canadians were similar to mine because of the marginalization and intersectional discrimination they have experienced throughout their lives. As it was for me, education as an institution seemed unattainable because of Blackness, disability, and discrimination. The intersection of the identities of Blackness and disability, and its impact on education, has long been a research interest of mine. The challenges facing Black students with disabilities suggests that an examination of a similar population in universities would be useful. The focus has been not only to formulate the theoretical characteristics of Blackness and disability in the university setting but also to analyze its practical implications.

In this book, I explore how Black undergraduate and graduate students with disabilities navigate the everyday complexities of Blackness and disabilities in university life. The University of Toronto was the site of this investigation, though this book is not intended to be a criticism or analysis of this institution specifically. A qualitative investigation of the way university bureaucracy interacts with Blackness and disability, I draw from the experiences of 12 Black students with disabilities at this university who met the inclusion criteria and were willing to share their lived experiences when seeking accommodation with the Accessibility Services Office.

Acknowledgments

This book has been a remarkable journey for me and would not have been possible without the love and support of several people who dared me to dream. I am grateful for the support of my incomparable PhD thesis advisor, Dr. Tanya Titchkosky, who has provided me with critical insights, invaluable commitment, and dedication. Dr. Titchkosky's work in the field of Disability Studies at the Ontario Institute for Studies in Education (OISE) of the University of Toronto was integral to the performance of my project, and her words guided me at several times through this process. The success of this book is due in no small part to her as well. I cannot underscore enough how thankful I am for Dr. Titchkosky's guidance and unwavering support. I am extremely grateful to Dr. Rod Michalko for his invaluable advice, words of wisdom, encouragement, and guidance. His theoretical work on marginality and disability as a "cultural production" functioned as the guidepost for my work in this book.

    I would also like to extend my deepest gratitude to Dr. Thomas Mathien for sharing his invaluable knowledge and critical insights for the completion of this book. My book owes its greatest debts to the participants at the University of Toronto with whom I carried out this study. Your enthusiasm and candid insights in sharing your reflections and experiences have been integral to the completion of this book. Many thanks to Dr. Anne McGuire and Dr. Patricia Douglas for their critical insights and support. Your continued generosity in sharing your knowledge and expertise in the fields of equity studies and disability studies is greatly appreciated. I wish to express my deepest gratitude to those scholars and sources whose critical works in the various subject areas of the discipline have contributed to the foundation of this book. To name a few: Professor Sylvia Wynter, Stuart Hall, Professor Kimberlé Crenshaw, Frantz Fanon, Dr. Patricia Hill Collins, Dr. Katherine McKittrick, Dr. bell hooks, Professor Rosemarie Garland-Thomson, Dr. Paul Gilroy, Dr. Lennard Davis, and Dr. Judith Butler.

I appreciate the financial support I received from the Social Sciences and Humanities Research Council (SSHRC) for their doctoral fellowship. It was an essential element of my doctoral research. I would like to thank the Ontario Graduate Scholarships (OGS) for their consistent funding throughout my doctoral studies as well. I would especially like to extend my gratitude to Dr. Judy Grant, Dr. Jacqui Getfield, Dr. Michelle Bailey and Dr. Jacqui Spencer. Together, I feel that we were able to form a special bond that was based on learning in the fields of anti-racism studies and equity studies. The support of my friends was also essential to my success in this process. I must acknowledge, Dr. Kim Borden, Dr. Devon Healey, Dr. Nolan Fontaine, Kelly-Ann Miller, Anthony Bedward, Anthony Foster, Audrey Morris, Lindsay Foster, Vivian Leslie, Tony Hunter, Simone Beckford, Porter Renfro IV and Ronnie Lindsey for being there with me through the process of completing my book. Without their support, the completion of my project would have been significantly more emotionally challenging and difficult; thus, they were a great part of going through my process. In particular, I want to thank Linda Awuni, who has been a source of encouragement and inspiration to me. To everyone, mentioned and unmentioned, thank you for the role you played in achieving the completion of this book project.

Introduction

In Canada, accessing higher education remains a significant challenge for Black people because of the inequities of systemic racism. Prejudiced approaches to administration and teaching lead to a lack of comfort among Black students. Despite some efforts of higher education in Canada to combat anti-Black racism and promote equity and inclusion, Black students continue to face significant challenges and barriers that negatively impact their educational experience and well-being (Adams, 2020; Baruwa, 2023: Lawson, 2020; Walcott, 2018). Recently, social movements, which call for increased visibility in policy and practice, have exposed the widespread discrimination affecting social minorities (Dei, 2017; Douglas, 2022), making it clear that individuals with disabilities frequently experience the poor social determinants linked with the burden of Black people, with heightened connections between race and disability.

Scholars of Black studies argue that anti-Blackness continues to take on new forms under the guise of "progress" in equity, diversity, and inclusion initiatives in higher educational institutions (Nxumalo & Gitari, 2021; Walcott, 2018). Similarly, other studies have found that systemic anti-Black racism is prevalent in Ontario's colleges and universities and that they are failing Black students (Baker, 2019; Cameron & Jefferies, 2021; Dryden & Nnorom, 2021; Tomlinson et al., 2021). Bruce (2021) used his own experiences as a Black man with mental illness to unearth the history of the Black radical tradition. In his work, he explores the history of the psychiatric system and its connection to racism, illustrating how Black people are often harmed and dehumanized in the name of mental health. Connecting to broader issues of social and political injustice, Bruce argues that mental illness has been an integral element of Black radical creativity.

When Blackness and disability are present in the same body, as this book examines, adequate academic accommodations in the university become increasingly challenging to obtain. Agents of the university, such as staff and faculty, create barriers to accommodations by either ignoring the real needs of these students or by using microaggression in a way that discourages students from seeking the accommodations they require to be productive in the classroom. Erevelles (2019) underlined that disability is common in educational research and contexts. The author further illustrates that the depiction of women and children with disability on social and other media compete with other images of suffering, attracting the attention of the global audience. In these descriptions, disability seems synonymous with an abject vulnerability, becoming simultaneously visible in its capacity to trigger an effective response and invisible when social policy is expected to respond to the real material consequence of living with a disability (Erevelles, 2019; Harris, 2021).

According to Vincent and Chiwandire (2019), Black students with disabilities consistently face barriers to accessing services and reasonable academic accommodations, preventing full participation in the university environment. For these students, academic accommodation is key to their thriving in the university setting, but they may fail to access the appropriate accommodations because the bureaucratic arrangements in the university themselves present a problem (Titchkosky, 2022). For these students, the lack of power to access appropriate accommodations is a constant challenge. In these cases, the only recourse is often an appeal to the system that has already judged their disability to be too insignificant to qualify for assistance. The experiences of these students highlight the crucial ways colonialism and structural inequities within the common perception of Blackness and disability continue to produce injustice in education, particularly in universities.

In this book, I draw on the theoretical insights of Kimberlé Crenshaw (1989) and Patricia Hill Collins (2015), whose work on the intersectionality of race and sex is central to my examination of the experiences of Black students with disabilities who face both institutional anti-Black racism and ableism in universities. In particular, I explore how students' identities of "Blackness" and "disability" are formed both at the administrative level and in everyday interactions in classrooms and how they navigate the quotidian complexities of university life. I use the word "disability" in this book in the context of the body of legislation, rules, and administrative interpretations thereof, not as a descriptor of the individual.

Accommodation matters greatly in the university because it is both pivotal to academic success and is beyond students' direct power to command. When the Black disabled student enters the university setting, they encounter and experience specific elements of the system. Blackness in the university system will typically lead to marginalization and fear because of how the system is structured. This book explores the nature of this marginalization and fear from the standpoint of the interactions students have with faculty and administrative staff. It also explores how this marginalization is magnified when students are both Black and disabled. Black students look at faculty and how they treat other students with similar characteristics when coming to understand their place in the university system. They understand that the university system creates marginalization and fear for other Black and disabled students; hence, this is the experience they will have too.

I aim to understand the nature of the marginalization these students experienced through their interaction with the bureaucracy of the university and its agents, such as staff members and faculty, whose decisions fortify the foundation of discrimination and injustice that they experience because of the inadequacy of the accommodation policies and procedures they enforce. According to the Ontario Human Rights Commission (OHRC, 2018), colleges and universities in Ontario,

Canada, are lagging behind in providing accessible academic accommodations to students with disabilities (p. 1).

I approach the theme of "disability as the problem in need of erasure" (Titchkosky & Michalko, 2017) by drawing a connection—via analogy—between the Black students' lived experiences reported for this research and the theoretical, scholarly discussion of the origins of normalcy and eugenic theories in nineteenth and twentieth century Europe and North America (Davis, 1995). From this perspective, we can understand how the theorizing of disability and Blackness enables us to critically engage with the discourses and practices of power that shape our everyday lives. I held that while we like to imagine ourselves as an inclusive society—and we would prefer to dismiss eugenics as a tragic and isolated aspect of history—there is a deep structural continuum connecting these movements and students' lived experiences in our educational environment. Students are often being "erased" from our education community and its social spaces in very real and effective ways.

I argue that the university systemizes marginalization through accommodation processes based on concepts of normalcy from which disability deviates. Black disabled students are essentially "invisible" to the bureaucracy. When they finally communicate their need for the accommodations, which the university is responsible for providing, the bureaucracy responds by resisting the students' efforts to achieve full inclusion and equity; that is, access to the same education that nondisabled students receive.

My investigation of Black disabled students' experiences at the University of Toronto deals with the visible and the invisible: the minority status of being racially Black as a visible trait and the often-invisible trait of disability, which cannot always be easily ascertained by outward inspection of the students. Many students interviewed had learning disabilities that they considered "invisible." Often the distinctions between visibility and invisibility is one of legal discernment. Black students are classified as "visible minorities" by the Government of Canada and by Canadian universities even when they represent a majority of the population in an area. In this research, I will argue that the idea of "invisibility" is useful (a) as a descriptive term, which is helpful for the political strategy of Black disabled students resisting the erasure of their future educational possibilities though unduly limited significations applied to their bodily identities in the university environment; and (b) in theoretical terms, which recognizes the limitations of models of the body, or bodily visibility, to fully represent all aspects of our complex and varied identities as human beings.

While we can understand the underlying need to address the multiple and complex perspectives of different forms of oppression, the recognition of this complexity should not—though it often does in practice—lead to overlooking the intersectional reality of Black disabled persons' experience of oppression. That is, Blackness and disability cannot be discussed outside contexts of power. As well, while disability is a phenomenon that is central to the experience of a significant portion of our population and is indeed a condition that we will all likely encounter as we age, it is also a topic that is an absent presence in our university discourse (Gill & Erevelles, 2017; Mitchell, 2017; Titchkosky et al., 2022). For example, in the daily lives of most of the academic community, Black students with disabilities probably seem invisible; the only sign of their presence being their Blackness and the "Under Repair" signs placed on disability access elevators, mobility ramps, or bathrooms around the university.

While Black and disabled people have been fighting for generations against systemic institutional discrimination, the struggle for *students* with disabilities is only beginning. There is a need to render this invisible population visible and foreground its needs in public discourse in a way that it is not at present. In fact, the same issues (e.g., equity, integration, access, inclusion) that animated the old civil rights movement have been renewed in the contemporary struggles of Black students with disabilities. As was the case with the civil rights movement, it is necessary to confront the policymaking elites to develop the means to address the needs of the student population with disabilities.

Of course, *Blackness* is not a disability, and this book approaches Blackness and disability from the standpoint that there is a unique phenomenon at play when a student is both Black and disabled. This phenomenon is multirelational in nature, and the marginalization, discrimination, and injustice experienced by students taking part in this research cannot be understood by treating Blackness as a disability. I use the term *Blackness* in this book to refer primarily to people who are Black, African, and of African descent.

According to Matlon (2022), Blackness is influenced by one's dark skin; the darker one is, the easier it is to identify as Black, which is mediated by other factors such as social class, nationality, culture, or racism. In addition, Mapedzahama and Kwansah-Aidoo (2017) note that Blackness is not only a visible marker of identity but also a sociopolitical relationship and political ontology (p. 1), as I discuss in depth in Chapter 1. However, Blackness and disability together create a different experience from that of a student who is only Black or only disabled. I explore how, when Blackness and disability are both present in the same body, others treat the subject as inherently weak and looking for an opportunity to obtain access to services fraudulently.

My investigation uncovers the origin, nature, methods, and limits of the intrinsic discriminatory foundations of the power structure as it exists in Canadian society. The subjects of this investigation find themselves confronting the unraveling of the meaning of intersectionality by exposing the causal roots of the discriminatory institutionalized power structure and the historical progression of these social constructs that culminated in the current circumstances, as discussed in the following chapters. Where the first approach is the *why* of intersectionality, the second investigatory approach is the *how*, which seeks an explanation rather than a mere description of the social construct. Finally, the third approach examines the critical praxis of the discriminatory social construct and how it relates to the subject of social justice and resistance to the power structure and its inherent discrimination.

Collins (2015) stated that this third approach diverges from the scholarly inquiry into the examination of the discriminatory practices in a broader sense. While the first two approaches are looking at the *why* and *how*, this third approach asks *where*. This question asks about the locality in the social construct that provides a focal point for any resistance. It seeks a tangible manifestation of intersectionality, where the efforts of social justice and resistance can be applied to deconstruct the discriminatory power structure as it exists in the community the students in the research are members of by virtue of their Blackness and disability.

In considering the challenge of resisting this pervasive institutional power structure, I found one potential avenue for resistance in a quotation from hooks (1990), cited by Titchkosky and Michalko (2009, p. 6) in their work on normalcy and disability. Acknowledging the reality of the marginalization of people with disabilities, these scholars go on to note:

> hooks tells us "that ... margins have been both sites of repression and sites of resistance." ... hooks suggests that respecting the voices, lives, and events found at the margins of a society might be a way to begin to resist and remake the centre's norms.

The theoretical purchase of this approach lies in its ability to acknowledge that Black students with disabilities—as with other oppressed groups in our society—are not going to suddenly occupy the center of our culture. Indeed, even when members of these groups are scholars, writing significant texts and conducting research widely recognized in their academic communities as important, they can still be represented as marginalized objects.

As Titchkosky (2011) points out, bureaucratic policy and practices are used to manage accessibility and accommodations for students with disabilities. She further notes that "paradoxical power [is] to make disability an unmanageable state of exception in the University environment" (p. 10). For instance, several students who participated in this research noted that although the accessibility system is intended to meet the needs of students with disabilities, it appears to produce problems and barriers to accessing the services being offered.

Observations in interpretive research require understanding the experience of subjects and how they may have come to construct their reality in their social setting. In the case of university students, that setting includes their university. The institutional educational environment is one where students may access several different types of accommodations. For each student, the experience of access can be different, for a multitude of reasons. For the Black disabled students, this experience can be significantly different from what it is for a student who is middle-to-upper class, able-bodied, white, and who has not sought services. The Black disabled student must cope with how bureaucracy works to process students with disabilities (Titchkosky, 2022; Waterfield et al., 2018).

The stories of these students are crucial to understanding their distinct experience as accommodation seekers. As Christine, a fourth-year undergraduate arts and sciences student stated, "I have often felt stigmatized and marginalized by faculty members at the onset of disclosing my need for accommodation." The experience of seeking services can be revealed by what students say about how they feel when they seek the services offered by the university. An example here is the experience of a student who is disabled in such a way that they cannot walk without assistance and their efforts to work with student housing services to access services related to accommodations.

The question of the quality of services offered emerges because students are deterred from accessing services; they must decide if they are willing to face yet another discussion or another need to prove eligibility. As racialized students with a disability, the students in this research have made a demand for personhood through "ability" and "access" as they try to overcome the emotional trauma that results from their interface with these bureaucratic policies and practices. The research argues that these students not only have to worry about the everyday complexities of Blackness and disability in university life "but also about their future [education] within it" (Thomas-Long, 2010, p. 153).

Insights from both Césaire's (1972) "Between Colonizer and Colonized" and Titchkosky's (2011) *The Question of Access: Disability, Space, Meaning* help us to understand Black disabled students' experience of normalization and marginality by providing guideposts on how to theorize social oppression and control. Both social oppression and control are exemplified in varying forms of colonization and exclusion and are central concerns in the operation of educational institutions. Indeed, just as Césaire conceptualizes colonization in the form of conflicting narratives of the same reality—"They talk about … [but] I am talking about …" as exemplified in an interpretive third- and first-person interface—Titchkosky (2011) argues that the "fight for access ... is also an interpretive space" (p. 91).

This interpretive context in which divergent narratives contest with each other for epistemological control over our physical, social, and cognitive space within education also reproduces disability as a problem that education is already troubled by and needs to manage through cognitive and physical interpretations of the self in an interpretive community. In this book, I understand power as the capacity to control our perspective on the world and how we interpret it. My research aims to show the ways Accessibility Services—like Césaire's colonizers—would prefer that their point of view, their "facts," be accepted as the meaning of accessibility.

However, if we hold a prism to these "facts"—as proposed by the bureaucracy's policy and practices—what filters through from the point of view of the students may be very different interpretations, conceptualizations, or "facts": an interpretive space in which the meaning is ... access denied! It is therefore important to emphasize that the struggle for inclusion or the struggle against colonization and anti-Black racism involves a struggle for control over narrative, interpretation, and meaning, a challenge that goes to the heart of such struggles against oppression in all their myriad forms (Pieterse et al., 2023; Walcott, 2017).

The intersectionality of Blackness and disability in higher education has not been well understood to date. There is a marked lack of consideration concerning how higher education can incorporate theorizations on Blackness and disability into a pragmatic understanding and how to address these marginalized voices. This book examines the impact of academic accommodation policies and practices on Black disabled university students' lived experiences. I pay close attention to a range of discourses on Blackness and disability that shape our understanding of the intersectionality of marginalization that Black students with disabilities experience in the university bureaucratic system. The following three research questions are the focus of this book:

- How are the categories of Blackness and disability constructed through university academic accommodation policy texts?

- How do these categories impact Black students who negotiate marginalized spaces within the university?
- How can a critical understanding of Blackness and disability be used to better inform educational policies and practices?

The aim of the book extends beyond simply examining the experiences of Black students with disabilities to explore how the two identities complement each other. For instance, are the challenges facing students who are both Black and disabled more than the sum of their parts? Accordingly, how should the intersectionality between the two identity categories be addressed?

I also consider the possible implications of theoretical research on Blackness and disability for practical implementations in higher education settings. While this book examines some of the challenges faced by Black students with disabilities at the University of Toronto, it also inquiries into the effects of academic accommodation practices by looking at how Black students with disabilities negotiate these accommodations in the university's bureaucratic system. However, to be identified as Black and disabled in the university environment is to face a host of difficulties. My research demonstrates how these difficulties and consequent marginalizing discrimination are normalized within and by the very university systems that explicitly aim to ameliorate them.

The findings of this research support this proposition: faculty appear to require greater proof of disability from Black disabled students than from others. It is essential to confront this injustice. One value of this research is in articulating the dimensions of the problem and proposing ways the issue could be addressed.

Discursive Intersectionality Framework

This book employs a novel, discursive intersectionality framework (Collins, 2015; Crenshaw, 1989) to explore the shared experiences of Black students with disabilities at the University of Toronto. This framework attends to the bureaucratic policies and practices that the 12 participants noted were deployed in their encounters with administrative personnel and university faculty when seeking academic accommodations.

Using this discursive framework, this book considers the intersection between Blackness and disability and how it relates to the bureaucratic policies and practices that organize students in the university setting. Critical analysis demonstrates the importance of considering how students' bodies are written upon and read through the language of Blackness and disability in educational institutions. I draw on various theories to illuminate the ways students navigate the everyday complexities of Blackness and disability in university life; however, these theories are not complete, revealing a gap in current understandings of the intersection of Blackness and disability in higher education. Filling this knowledge gap will aid in understanding how administrative policy in the university setting impacts the lives of Black disabled students. The foundation of this gap lies in an overall approach to education that continues to be shaped by colonial elements.

To examine these effects, including racialization, normalization, and subjugation, requires a delineation of the common experiences of students to provide insight into life at the university. Showing how the identities of Black and disabled intersect may be necessary to unsettle the stable Blackness-disability discourses and practices that are apparent in public, regulated spaces (Adjei, 2018; Banks et al., 2022; Erevelles, 2019; Pickens, 2021; Watermeyer & Swartz, 2023; Wynter, 2003). In this book, I approach Blackness and disability from the standpoint that there is a unique phenomenon at play when a student is both Black and disabled.

One aspect of this book examines how the legacies of colonialism continue to impact Black university students' experiences. I use critical theoretical approaches drawn from a Black studies perspective to disrupt how the process of colonialism operates in educational institutions. A discursive approach allows interrogation of the problem of colonialism, its pedagogies, and the cultural production of marginalized students. It is often very difficult for Black disabled students to navigate the very systems designed to accommodate their needs as individuals. In this book, I show how institutionalized accommodation procedures relegate students to an alternative status despite the stated goals of the university and civic policies to equalize avenues of opportunity.

Moreover, it is important, within the context of a study informed by a critique of anti-Black racism, to recognize the struggle against structural inequalities based on racial categories in educational institutions. The reoccurring theme of incredulity about the need for accommodations and the inequity of expectations of students from racial minorities (Titchkosky, 2022; Walcott, 2018) can be accounted for by this book.

In analyzing the power structure of the university and its Accessibility Services office, the mono-system's analysis of racism or ableism each provides an incomplete account of the social inequalities. A mono-systematic analysis of racism, as used in this context, refers to the approach to the examination or study of racism where race is isolated as the singular social formation and knowledge project based on which people are discriminated against and abused. A mono-systems analysis of racism exclusively focuses on racism, its mechanisms, structures, and impacts without also considering how other social formations and knowledge projects, such as ableism, sexism, classism, and homophobia, intersect to compound the experiences of the racially abused individuals (Collins, 2015, p. 5). A mono-systems analysis of racism is oblivious to the fact that various social structures and cultural representations deeply intertwine and interconnect leading to complex social inequalities. While it's not in doubt that race or Blackness itself has significant ontological, epistemological, and axiological implications on how an individual perceives themselves and relate with other people in social settings (Collins et al., 2021, p. 694; Mulderink, 2023, p. 10), various social structures that define their identity are also relevant and these may only be comprehensively conceptualized through the lens of intersectionality. Collins (2015) notes the true complexity of inequality in social relationships:

> Intersectionality can build on this foundation by moving beyond a mono-categorical focus on racial inequality to encompass multiple forms of inequality that are organized via a similar logic. As an initial step, this framework can be applied to other social formations and knowledge projects that reproduce inequality, for example, social formations of patriarchy, capitalism, heterosexism, and their characteristic knowledge projects. Yet, intersectionality

goes farther than this mono-system analysis, introducing a greater level of complexity into conceptualizing inequality. (p. 5)

Collins went on to describe the forms of knowledge projects using the intersectionality framework, noting that there were typically two primary investigatory approaches in describing this social construct. The first is intersectionality as a field of study, as the object of the investigation, making explanatory determinations of *why* this social construct exists and how it fits into the prevailing power relationships. Ultimately, this approach makes the concept of intersectionality the focus of the inquiry by extrapolating the facets of the power structure and discriminatory nature of society. The second approach uses the concept of intersectionality as an analytical strategy, where the concept is employed to render new knowledge of the social world in which these power structures and discriminatory patterns are allowed to exist, foment, and reinforce the power structure paradigm.

I delineate the bureaucratic policy system to understand how Black disabled students are expected to negotiate their learning experiences. As the students face the problems of accommodation and educational practices in the university environment, the university as a social institution manages and maintains the provision of what it deems to be accessible academic accommodations for students with disabilities.

Universities espouse working to "eliminate" problems such as systemic discrimination; however, they continue to fail to do so, especially in the ways they deal with students who are marginalized in complex and compounding ways (e.g., through race, Blackness, disability, class, gender, sexuality, and other forms of marginality). For those bureaucrats who have seen limited changes in policies designed to address the problems of academic accommodations, those changes may appear to be sufficient because any change will feel significant given how systemic shifts are perceived by those inside the bureaucracy. For Black students, however, these have been inadequate.

This research tries to understand the issue of intersectional discrimination and marginality and the way bureaucratic elements such as academic policy have continued to support this discrimination. The intersectionality of Blackness and disability is an under-investigated reality of daily life for a significant segment of the student and provincial population. In the following chapters, I explore some of the challenges faced by Black students with disabilities in Canadian universities and discuss ways to address these challenges, particularly anti-Blackness and marginalization.

McCall (2009) considers "the complexity of intersectionality" as an apt framework for, and exploration of, inherently complex social relations and finds that "research practice mirrors the complexity of social life" (p. 49). The desire for the simplification of social constructs such as Blackness and disability to facilitate the explanation of a social phenomenon can be frustrated by the very nature of the complexities of society. I investigate precursors to the social constructs we know today and the development of the power structure that provides the pillars on which discrimination rests. McCall recounts three methodological approaches to addressing the issue of complexity in the investigation of intersectionality, which I integrate into the intersectionality framework of this book.

The first methodological approach related by McCall (2009) is *anticategorical complexity*, which seeks to deconstruct analytical categories, recognizing that society is too irreducibly complex to readily facilitate simplification in broad terms. Instead, it isolates and investigates each nuanced aspect of the social framework. This approach rejects categorizing society and is at the far end of the analytical spectrum. The second methodological approach lies in the middle ground and is deemed *intracategorical complexity*. This approach focuses on a broad categorization that is intellectually comfortable for investigations while maintaining a certain amount of skepticism for the categorization paradigm. It is useful for the investigations into "people whose identity crosses the boundaries of traditionally constructed groups" (p. 50).

This middle ground of categorization is contrasted with the third methodological approach of *intercategorical complexity*, which creates comfortable categories that fall in line with traditional forms of methodological approach. McCall notes that this "provisional" categorization in research constitutes a methodological approach. It employs methods of defining categories to facilitate research rather than seeking to allow the investigatory process to evolve independently.

This discursive approach examines all aspects of the experience of Black students with disabilities at the University of Toronto. The intersectionality approach provides an alternative to a mono-system approach, where multiple inequalities of the oppressed and excluded are taken into account in the study of their marginalization and normalcy, especially within university settings. It brings to the fore how the university power structure perpetuates inequality and discrimination in all its varied forms.

The issue of disability in the university environment is one of the two key pillars of this investigation and is part of the larger action of the university bureaucracy that removes the student's individuality and seeks to "classify" or "categorize" them with an identity dominated by their disability. Titchkosky (2010) noted about the power of the university's bureaucratic policies and practices:

> The global process of bureaucratizing embodiment recommends that it is fair, morally correct, legally efficacious, or even tacitly neutral to regard disability as a condition attached to some people while disregarding the ways disability is differentially conceptualized around the world. (p. 3)

Extending Titchkosky's analysis of bureaucratic arrangements in educational institutions, my research examines these practices and discourses through a critical lens to explore the complexities of students' experiences within the institutional setting. The interaction between students and administration serves to diminish the former's personhood. Students are framed in a manner that the bureaucratic apparatus can recognize as *clients*. While some modicum of accommodation is granted through routine or systematic practices, bureaucracies do so with little measure of the success or failure of the students as individuals in the classroom environment.

From a practical standpoint, one objective of this research is to lead administration and faculty to consider how the bureaucracy has been a problem for students who have been marginalized in complex and compounding ways (e.g., through race, Blackness, disability, class, gender and sexuality, and other forms of marginality) and determine how problems can be addressed.

My analysis of the data used for this book is guided by principles of intersectionality. This framework goes beyond the measuring of outcomes and beyond any single dimension of a lone variable. This intersectionality points us toward the multifaceted relationship between a complex social location and the structural features including inequalities of public policy. The analysis takes into account the interconnection and intersection of various social variables such as sexism, homophobia, ableism, and anti-Blackness, and their correlation with the notable institutionalized racialized prejudices. It focuses on members of an oppressed group that dwell in the complexity of the interaction between these social factors (Bindley et al., 2023; Collins & Bilge, 2020; Crenshaw, 1989; Hankivsky, 2012). The accessibility requirements of the university at which the students in this research study were enrolled are a matter of public policy and provincial law implemented at the university level, the administration of such is affected by Accessibility Services as well as professors and teaching staff.

In addition to considering the discursive bureaucratic policies and practices that affect Black students with disabilities, my research was also guided by sociologist Dorothy Smith's (2005) writings on institutional ethnography. They provide insight into the students' personal experiences as a response to the institutional context. University bureaucracy in and of itself can impede the academic performance of the student:

> If we take up the realities of students' work lives as the actual situations in which they produce tests and assignments for the instructor to grade, we can see that grades may be strongly affected by the number of courses a student is taking and hence the kind of pressure of time and anxiety that hits at the end of term …. Physical disabilities transform the work of getting to the library, to class, to materials, and so on. All these matters take time; traveling from home to the university takes time. The work of getting to class, to the library, to making what's to be studied into a form in which it is accessible, dealing with the university bureaucracy—all of these also take time, and all of these take longer for a student who's disabled. Time deployed in ways such as these diminish what is available for intensive study and writing or preparation for tests; less time spent in study and preparation means lower grades. (p. 148)

The observation of the time aspect and the interaction with university bureaucracy was key in my interviews with the students. Following the provisos of the discursive bureaucratic policies and practices framework, my research focused on the experiences of students both in the classroom setting and in negotiating the bureaucracy of the Accessibility Services office while pursuing reasonable academic accommodations necessitated by their disability and guaranteed in both statute and policy.

Racism and ableism function both separately and together, leading to disqualification and tokenization of Black people with disabilities. Mulderink (2023) points out that a Black disabled student is not a typical client at the disability resource centers and is therefore not treated like the rest of the students (p. 26). This is best understood from the base understanding of disability resource centers as predominantly white spaces. Further, the white spaces' conception of disability is inclined towards a medical model as opposed to a social model. Effectively, a disabled person is seen as a sick, deficient, and impaired individual who requires fixing by diagnosing, treating, and curing the impairment (López et al., 2017; Michalko & Goodley, 2023; Sandahl, 2004; Titchkosky, 2020). A social model on the other hand, sees disability as unique and sociological in the sense that it located the disability outside the individual by focusing on the societal barriers that contribute to the individual's disability. It is noteworthy that Canadian educational institutions lack "disability spaces" that would lead to better and more meaningful accommodation of disabled persons. Disability spaces, the literature notes, would enable individuals to develop a sense of belonging. To the extent that the educational institutions are "white spaces" and lack "disability spaces," the intersectionality of racism and ableism crystallizes in the experiences of the Black disabled students (McRuer, 2008, p. 69; Mulderink, 2023, p. 28).

Annamma (2018) observes that the intersectionality of ableism and racism in the educational context manifests in the fact that people of color with disabilities face significant economic challenges that hinder their educational performance (p. 78). For instance, they are often placed in particular education environments due to economic deficiencies. Second, the households of people of color with a disability may not have the financial means to access the learning disability diagnosis that would enable them to gauge their suitability to access mainstream classrooms with non-disabled students (Mulderink, 2023, p. 64). This factor compounds their inequality and exclusion. Therefore, even in instances where people of color with disabilities are identified as transabled, their circumstances hinder their access to disability support services provided by educational institutions. For this reason, Mulderink (2023) concludes that even the policies that are prima facie intended to promote inclusivity and equality for all people uphold whiteness in inherently white spaces (p. 64). Moreover, it is reported that Black people with a disability are more likely to experience criminalization of disability compared to their white counterparts. Specifically, the fact of disability may itself be construed as a prima facie indication of a lack of discipline or a consequence of defiance (Mulderink, 2023, p. 64). This may inform the various institutional approaches to discipline practices for disabled students where they are overtly or covertly discriminated against based on their race. Such disciplinary practices may, for instance, include restricted access to disability resource centers.

We find this, for example, in the way American exceptionalism is manifest in various educational institutions in the United States. American exceptionalism is the cultural ideology positing that the American nation is inherently exceptional with a unique, solemn responsibility to transform the world through its global leadership. It assumes the superiority of the American state (Walt, 2024, para 2). For instance, some educational policies include students regarded as having impairments (whether or not they had physical impairments) in Accessibility Resource centers (Annamma, 2018). This has the danger of obscuring and ignoring the rights of disabled students. These experiences of Black people with disabilities indicate that as much as educational institutions throw around words like diversity, equity, and inclusion in their policies and practices, these ideals are not necessarily reflected in the concrete policies and practices. There are manifest ambiguities in the construction and application of the policies, a fact that may perhaps be attributed to the whiteness of the educational spaces and the underlying notions of white supremacy and ableism.

In this book, the intersectionality of Blackness and disability is analogous to Crenshaw's examination of race and sex in that the dual status of racial minority and disability are distinct sources of historical discrimination and subjugation of the individual. Thus, each alone would provide ample material for an investigation into discriminatory practices and inherent biases at a university or the accessibilities services hierarchy. However, the intersection of these two frameworks, when viewed through the lens of discursive bureaucratic policies and practices, provides a unique perspective into the common experiences of the students and the subject population they represent. Their experiences juxtapose the stated goals of equality in both racial and accommodation policies with their practical applications in the university's educational environment. It is important to note that the legal and policy requirements of equality, as examined within these two theoretical frameworks, in practice fall short of their lofty expectations. The practical experiences of students, as documented by this research, reveals an environment far removed from the expectation of equality.

To answer the question "How does a university's academic accommodation practices and policies impact lives of Black disabled students," I employed a qualitative methodology using open-ended interviews that permitted the free expression of opinions and feelings. In the potentially prejudicial role as both researcher and member of the selected group, it was all the more important that I maintain impartiality while presenting an element of empathy, as many of the personal histories and experiences of the students were replete with trauma; however, difficult anecdotes were essential to my inquiry.

Thus, the research data underpinning my conclusions in this book are derived from interviews with 12 Black students (both undergraduate and graduates) who self-identified as having a disability, representing a diverse cross-section of the targeted population. The majority were women, with three men participants and nine women. The breakdown of the participants can be found in Appendix B. All participants were given pseudonyms; none of the names in this book represent the real names of actual study participants. I asked each of these students open-ended questions to elicit a response and was surprised at their honesty and candor. The institutionalization of a power structure under the auspice of assisting students with disabilities was at the crux of these questions (see Appendix A).

Black students who face discrimination or disability labeling often face disadvantages in schooling, which inevitably reproduces inequality. This research engages critical and interpretive methods and theories within sociology as well as Black studies and disability studies to illuminate the ways students navigate everyday complexities of Blackness and disability in university life. By examining student experiences, this book highlights how accommodation, as a facet of access, "performs" or "enacts" inequality.

The use of student experiences in this book runs parallel to Crenshaw's (1989) use of court rulings in her critical comments on previous approaches to antidiscrimination, feminist theory, and antiracist politics. Crenshaw discusses the intersection of race and gender, noting that there has been a lack of consideration in society for the experiences of Black women. In general, the stigma carried by Black people is such that their experiences are deemed less trustworthy than the experiences of white people. Consequently, there is a stigma that follows the Black experience. This stigma contributes to the difficulties that persist in the lives of Black people, where their lack of privilege makes it difficult to gain access to services. McKittrick (2011) noted:

> A Black sense of place is not a steady, focused, and homogeneous way of seeing and being in place, but rather a set of changing and differential perspectives that are illustrative of, and therefore remark upon, legacies of normalized racial violence that calcify, but do not guarantee, the denigration of black geographies and their inhabitants. (p. 950)

The sense of place identified by McKittrick, for the purposes of my research, is not a physicality but rather a social pattern in the university that the established power structure seeks to maintain. The plantation mentality is an effect of an entrenched social pattern: "The plantation evidences an uneven colonial–racial economy that, while differently articulated across time and place, legalized Black servitude while simultaneously sanctioning Black placelessness and constraint" (McKittrick, 2011, p. 948). The university and its Accessibility Services maintain a power structure and social construct that reflect, and reproduce, the slave plantation mentality with control over the labor force for the benefit of the owners.

My research draws on the scholarly literature on race, Blackness, identity, equity, and the normalization of marginality that Black disabled

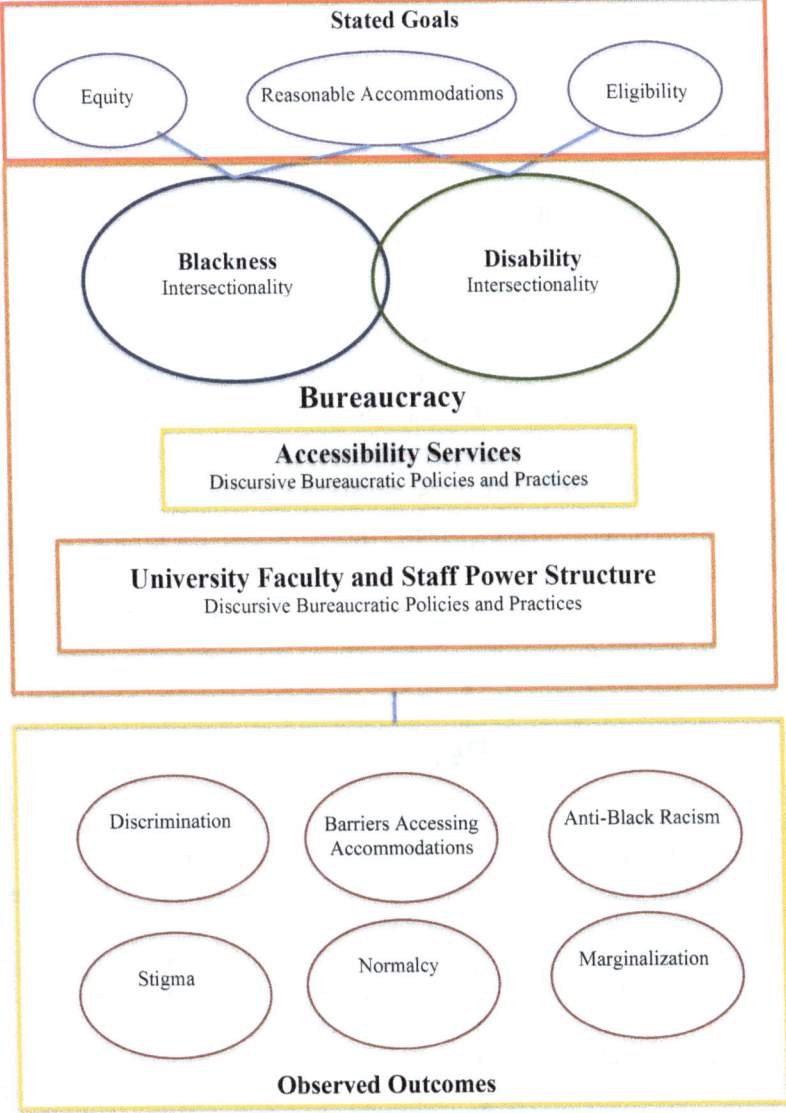

Figure 1.1. Blackness and Disability Research Flowchart

students experience, as well as the nature of discursive bureaucratic accommodation practices impacting these students. Scholars in Black studies and disability studies seem to agree that racialized people have differential experiences in education, including in higher education (Basile & Black, 2019; Cummings & Mohabir, 2022; Dolmage, 2017; Morales, 2021). While Black and disability studies theorists all share an underlying preoccupation with how identity and the self are deployed and used by elites as strategies of discursive power and political control, I believe that extending this analysis to Blackness and disability in higher education opens critical space to further explore the modalities of power and domination.

Figure 1.1 highlights an in-depth understanding of Black students' common experiences at their university. The flowchart shown is a diagrammatic depiction of the 14 components of intersectionality and discursive bureaucratic policies and practices. The chart begins with the stated goals of creating access, reasonable accommodations, and eligibility for Black students with disabilities. Reasonable accommodations are a focus for both Blackness and disability; however, equity is only focused upon for Black students, while eligibility is only focused on for the disabled. This leaves Black *and* disabled students at a point of intersectionality. The outcomes observed are discrimination, stigma, normalcy, and barriers when accessing accommodations, anti-Black racism, and marginalization.

References

Adams, T. L. (2020). *How to be an antiracist*. by Ibram X. Kendi. *Journal of Communication Inquiry, 45*(2), 199–201. https://doi.org/10.1177/0196859920961032.

Adjei, P. B. (2018). The (em)bodiment of blackness in a visceral anti-Black racism and ableism context. *Race Ethnicity and Education, 21*(3), 275–287.

Annamma, S. (2018). *The pedagogy of pathologization: Dis/abled girls of color in the school-prison nexus* (1st ed.). Retrieved from: https://www.routledge.com/The-Pedagogy-of-Pathologization-Disabled-Girls-of-Color-in-the-School-prison-Nexus/Annamma/p/book/9781138696907.

Baker, L. A. (2019). *Normalizing marginality: A critical analysis of blackness and disability in higher education* [Unpublished doctoral dissertation]. University of Toronto.

Banks, J., Smith, P., & Charington Neal, D. (2022). Identity politics: Exploring DisCrit's potential to empower activism and collective resistance. In S. A. Annamma, B. A. Ferri, & D. J. Connor (Eds.), *DisCrit expanded: Reverberations, ruptures, and inquiries* (pp. 96–111). Teacher's College Press.

Baruwa, I. (2023). Black Students' *Academic Experiences at Canadian Universities: A Methodological Literature Review*. Retrieved from https://papers.ssrn.com/sol3/papers.cfm?abstract_id=4445673.

Basile, V., & Black, R. (2019). They hated me till I was one of the "good ones": Toward understanding and disrupting the differential racialization of undergraduate African American STEM majors. *The Journal of Negro Education, 88*(3), 379–390.

Bindley, K., Lewis, J., Travaglia, J., & DiGiacomo, M. (2023). Bureaucracy and burden: An intersectionality-based policy analysis of social welfare policy with consequences for carers of people with life-limiting illness. *Palliative Medicine, 37*(4), 543–557.

Bruce, L. M. (2021). *How to go mad without losing your mind*. https://doi.org/10.1515/9781478012429.

Cameron, E. S., & Jefferies, K. (2021). Anti-Black racism in Canadian education: A call to action to support the next generation. *Healthy Populations Journal, 1*(1).

Césaire, A. (1972). *Discourse on colonialism*. Trans. J. Pinkham. Monthly Review Press.

Collins, P. H. (2015). Intersectionality's definitional dilemmas. *Annual Review of Sociology*, 41, 1–20.

Collins, P. H., & Bilge, S. (2020). *Intersectionality* (2nd ed.). Polity Press.

Collins, P. et al. (2021). Intersectionality as critical social theory, 20, pp. 690–725. Retrieved from: https://doi.org/10.1057/s41296-021-00490-0.

Crenshaw, K. (1989). Demarginalizing the intersection of race and sex: A black feminist critique of antidiscrimination doctrine, feminist theory and antiracist politics. *University of Chicago Legal Forum*, 139–167.

Cummings, R., & Mohabir, N. (2022). Protests and pedagogy: The legacies of Caribbean student resistance and the Sir George Williams protest, Montreal 1969. *TOPIA: Canadian Journal of Cultural Studies, 44*, 1–24.

Davis, L. J. (1995). *Enforcing normalcy: Disability, deafness, and the body*. Verso Books.

Dei, G. J. (2017). [Re]framing blackness and black solidarities through anti-colonial and decolonial prisms: An introduction. *Reframing Blackness and Black Solidarities through Anti-Colonial and Decolonial Prisms*, 1–30. https://doi.org/10.1007/978-3-319-53079-6_1.

Dolmage, J. T. (2017). *Academic ableism: Disability and higher education*. University of Michigan Press.

Douglas, D. (2022). At the crossroads, Black disabled lives do matter: Intersections of race and disability in special education. *Johns Hopkins University, 3*(1).

Dryden, O., & Nnorom, O. (2021). Time to dismantle systemic anti-Black racism in medicine in Canada. *CMAJ, 193*(2), E55–E57.

Erevelles, N. (2019). "Scenes of subjection" in public education: Thinking intersectionally as if disability matters. *Educational Studies, 55*(6), 592–605. https://doi.org/10.1080/00131946.2019.1687481.

Gill, M., & Erevelles, N. (2017). The absent presence of Elsie Lacks: Hauntings at the intersection of race, class, gender, and disability. *African American Review, 50*(2), 123–137.

Hankivsky, O. (Ed.). (2012). *An intersectionality-based policy analysis framework.* Institute for Intersectionality Research and Policy, Simon Fraser University.

Harris, J. (2021, July 26). *Reckoning with race and disability.* SSRN. https://papers.ssrn.com/sol3/papers.cfm?abstract_id=3878540.

hooks, b. (1990). Marginality as a site of resistance. *Out There: Marginalization and Contemporary Cultures, 4,* 341–343.

Lawson, E. S. (2020). Anti-Black racism on the sidelines: The limits of "listening sessions" to address institutional racism at Canadian universities. *Canadian Review of Sociology, 57*(3), 491–495.

Mapedzahama, V., & Kwansah-Aidoo, K. (2017). Blackness as burden? The lived experience of Black Africans in Australia. *Sage Open, 7*(3). https://doi.org/10.1177/2158244017720483

Matlon, J. (2022). *A man among other men: The crisis of Black masculinity in racial capitalism.* Cornell University Press. https://doi.org/10.1515/9781501762871

McCall, L. (2009). The complexity of intersectionality. In E. Grabham, D. Cooper, J. Krishnadas, & D. Herman (Eds.), *Intersectionality and beyond: Law, power and the politics of location* (pp. 49–76). Routledge-Cavendish.

McKittrick, K. (2011). On plantations, prisons, and a black sense of place. *Social & Cultural Geography, 12*(8), 947–963.

McRuer, R. (2008). Crip theory. Cultural signs of queerness and disability. *Scandinavian Journal of Disability Research, 10*(1), 67, 69.

Michalko, R., & Goodley, D. (2023). *Letters with Smokie: Blindness and More-than-Human Relations.* University of Manitoba Press.

Mitchell, D.T. (2017). Disability, diversity, and diversion: Normalization and avoidance in higher education. In *Disability, Avoidance and the Academy* (pp. 9–20). Routledge.

Morales, E. (2021). "Beasting" at the battleground: Black students responding to racial microaggressions in higher education. *Journal of Diversity in Higher Education, 14*(1), 72.

Mulderink, C. (2023). The intersection of racism and ableism in disability support services. *Communication ETDs* [Preprint]. Retrieved from: https://digitalrepository.unm.edu/cj_etds/156.

Nxumalo, F., & Gitari, W. (2021). Introduction to the special theme on responding to anti-Blackness in science, mathematics, technology and STEM education. *Canadian Journal of Science, Mathematics and Technology Education, 21,* 226–231.

Ontario Human Rights Commission. (OHRC). (2018). *Ableism rife in Ontario schools, rights commission says.* CBC.com. Retrieved from https://www.cbc.ca/news/canada/ottawa/students-disabilities-discrimination-ontario-1.4803793.

Pickens, T. A. (2021). Blackness and disability: The remix. *CLA Journal, 64*(1), 3–10.

Pieterse, A. L., Lewis, J. A., & Miller, M. J. (2023). Dismantling and eradicating anti-Blackness and systemic racism. *Journal of counseling psychology, 70*(3), 235.

Sandahl, C. (2004). Black man, blind man: Disability identity politics and performance. *Theatre Journal*, 56(4), 579–602.
Smith, D. E. (2005). *Institutional ethnography: A sociology for people*. AltaMira Press.
Thomas-Long, R. (2010). *The politics of exclusion in graduate education*. Peter Lang.
Titchkosky, T., & Michalko, R. (2009). *Rethinking normalcy: A disability studies reader*. Canadian Scholars' Press.
Titchkosky, T. (2010). The not-yet-time of disability in the bureaucratization of university life. *Disability Studies Quarterly*, 30(3/4). http://dsq sds.org/article/view/1295/1331.
Titchkosky, T. (2011). *The question of access: Disability, space, meaning*. University of Toronto Press.
Titchkosky, T. (2020). The cost of counting disability: Theorizing the possibility of a non-economic remainder. *Critical Readings in Interdisciplinary Disability Studies: (Dis) Assemblages*, 25–40.
Titchkosky, T. (2022). University inclusion practices—re-encountering the status quo: An interpretive approach. *Journal of Disability Studies in Education (online)*, 3(1), 102–124. https://doi.org/10.1163/25888803-bja10017.
Titchkosky, T., & Michalko, R. (2017). The body as a problem of individuality: A phenomenological disability studies approach. In *Disability, Space, Architecture* (pp. 67–294). Routledge. https://doi.org/10.4324/9781315560076-10.
Titchkosky, T., Cagulada, E., DeWelles, M., & Gold, E. (Eds.). (2022). *DisAppearing: Encounters in disability studies*. Canadian Scholars Press.
Tomlinson, A., Mayor, L., & Baksh, N. (2021, February 24). Being Black on campus: Why students, staff and faculty say universities are failing them. *CBC News*. https://www.cbc.ca/news/canada/anti-black-racism-campus-university-1.5924548
Vincent, L., & Chiwandire, D. (2019). Funding and inclusion in higher education institutions for students with disabilities. *African Journal of Disability*, 8(1), 1–12.
Walcott, R. (2017). Time for white left to speak up on anti-Black racism. *Now Magazine Toronto*. https://nowtoronto.com/news/time-for-white-left-to-speak-up/.
Walcott, R. (2018). Against social justice and the limits of diversity: Or Black people and freedom. In *Toward what justice?* (pp. 85–99). Routledge.
Walt, S. M. (2024). The Myth of American Exceptionalism. *Foreign Policy*, 20 June. Retrieved from: https://foreignpolicy.com/2011/10/11/the-myth-of-american-exceptionalism/ (Accessed: 19 June 2024).
Waterfield, B., Beagan, B. B., & Weinberg, M. (2018). Disabled academics: A case study in Canadian universities. *Disability & Society*, 33(3), 327–348.
Watermeyer, B., & Swartz, L. (2023). Disability and the problem of lazy intersectionality. *Disability & Society*, 38(2), 362–366.
Wynter, S. (2003). Unsettling the coloniality of being/power/truth/freedom: Towards the human, after man, its overrepresentation—An argument. *CR: The New Centennial Review*, 3(3), 257–337.

Part I

Identity: The Visible vs the Invisible

The idea of identity is becoming increasingly complex. These complexities are present both in how academic study is performed and how people see themselves and the groups they belong to. Alcoff (2006) discussed identity as fluctuating with the way people see the differences between themselves and others and noted that this difference is supported through academic literature as demographic elements such as gender become important factors influencing the nature of current research and how the implications of this research are understood.

Alcoff (2006) argued that this is also a part of how we understand politics, social status, and economic strata. These differences become part of how people perceive their identity, and they can become both barriers to understanding and the basis for how groups of people marginalize one another. Marks of identity will signal to other people that there are significant differences between themselves and others and determine whether or not they will support those others.

Identity politics can be read as implicated in creating categories of understanding that fit into the dominant culture's agenda of creating an "other" existing outside of the norm (Rajchman, 1995). One of the major claims of post-modern thinking is that identity should be called into question as a stable category of being and representation (Rajchman, 1995). This remains a prominent critique that has affected several areas of social and political thought and has also impacted how we talk about identity politics, especially in terms of gender and race.

There is an argument that a subject's identity has been "overrepresented," meaning that the conception of what it is to be human is itself a product of Western and bourgeois thinking, which Wynter (1994) defined as the "coloniality of being," where dominating classes and powers have decided what it is to be an autonomous person with full rights. In that case, our struggles with representing race, Blackness, disability, class, and gender are bound up in the history of oppression that has been propagated by colonizing and often Western powers.

Wynter grapples with the complexity of the relationship between the body and the socially constructed self. Wynter (2003) theorizes that the "body" serves as a cultural "anchor" for the self in terms of identity, suggesting that "gender … has a biogenetically determined anatomical differential correlate onto which each culture's system of gender oppositions can be anchored" (p. 264). Interestingly, however, she contends that while "race" is a "purely invented construct" racial identity—given this "anchor"—is not.

It is understandably difficult to grapple with issues relating to the bio-genesis of the self (Cooley, 1902; Davis, 1995; Fanon, 1963). However, Wynter's comments above highlight not only the basis of this modern labeling or construction of the self in discourse but also the challenges of interrogating or subverting these processes. For example, in Western countries today, it would be at most a minority view that Black and disabled people were subhuman—or inferior—due to their physical/biological characteristics. Yet, in those same societies, the struggles for civil and disability rights persist due in large measure to the success of authoritarian forces at redeploying their discursive capabilities in subtle ways.

The character of subjectivity is a deep philosophical question and is connected to one's self or related self-governance of one's own actions in social contexts (Foucault, 1994, p. 90). In the context of the investigation of Blackness and disability, it relates to how students care for themselves in a university setting with regards to their disability and state of being a racial body. It speaks to the action that the students take to exist in an environment where they are subject to two disadvantages perceived by society: the fact that the students are Black, a racial minority historically discriminated against in terms of educational opportunities, and live with a disability that also hinders their performance in a university setting. It goes beyond mere adaptation and accommodation; subjectivity speaks to the specific actions the students take to facilitate their university education career.

Identity is an important individual and social phenomenon. For Black individuals with a disability, it is important to examine how society contributes to the construction of identities and how this impacts both the way Black disabled persons see themselves and the way others see them—but also the ramifications of this for the way people see the types of assistance that are given to Black disabled students to support equity.

The paradoxical reality of Black people in predominantly white spaces is that they are hypervisible yet invisible at the same time. This may seem contradictory given that visible is the opposite of invisible. How is it possible to be visible yet invisible? Newton (2022) interviewed 25 undergraduate Black women at a university in the Midwestern United States. The data from these interviews demonstrate this paradoxical reality. It was reported that Black undergraduate women's marginalization was marked by their invisibility and hypervisibility (p. 165). They stated that because of their Blackness and gender, they were hypervisible, making them viable targets for microaggressions from white supremacists. Conversely, despite their hypervisibility, they were ignored and excluded from interactions with white students on the campus (Newton, 2022). In other words, Black women were hypervisible for the purposes of racial and sexist microaggressions but invisible within meaningful and respectful human interactions (Lopez, 2017, p. 11; Newton, 2022). This sums up the reality for Black people, who are deemed invisible in generic spaces. Their presence is erased and they are treated as though they do not exist, even when the conversation is supposed to benefit them. This invisibility manifests in the invalidation and subjugation of the community.

For instance, Black peoples' voices are ignored when raised against the microaggressions they are subjected to, whereas when the voices are such that they reinforce the white supremacist racial stereotype of Black backwardness, they are heard and seen. Another manifestation of this paradox is in the culture and practice of tokenism, where Black women are, for instance, employed not because of the acknowledgment of their competence and qualification but to enable the employer to tick a box of diversity and inclusivity (Newton, 2022, p. 166; Reiter & Reiter, 2020, p. 35). The combination of Blackness and gender help the employer give the impression that they are committed to gender equality and racial balance.

Newton (2022) states that from her study, which focused on microaggressions, she discovered that Black women's reality in predominantly white neighborhoods experiences micro invalidation and micro invisibility (p. 166). An example of the manifestation of this paradox is the narrative by one of the participants. She narrated an incident where she was walking alongside her ex-boyfriend on campus and was approached by a white student to join a student organization. While they were both senior marketing majors, the ex-boyfriend was ignored and uninvited, as though he was invisible (Newton, 2022, p. 170). Several similar instances were reported, which indicate some form of tokenism based on race and gender. This invisibility-hypervisibility paradox is not without tangible consequences. For example, Black students feel isolated and alienated, hence unable to establish meaningful interpersonal relationships with their white peers. This makes the Black students feel "seen as the unseen." In other words, Black people are seen for their Blackness, not their individuality. Mills (1998) argues that seeing racial minorities as only Black is not seeing them at all. They are deprived of their individuality and demeaned as human beings.

References

Alcoff, L. M. (2006). *Visible identities: Race, gender, and the self.* Oxford University Press.
Cooley, C. (1902). *Human nature and the social order.* Charles Scribner's Sons.
Davis, L. J. (1995). *Enforcing normalcy: Disability, deafness, and the body.* Verso Books.
Fanon, F. (1963). *The wretched of the earth.* Grove Press.

Foucault, M. (1994). Subjectivity and truth. In J. Faubion (Ed.), *Ethics: Subjectivity and truth* (pp. 87–92). New Press.

López, N. et al. (2017). Making the invisible visible: advancing quantitative methods in higher education using critical race theory and intersectionality. *Race Ethnicity and Education, 21*, pp. 1–28. Retrieved from: https://doi.org/10.1080/13613 324.2017.1375185.

Mills, C. (1998). *Blackness visible* (1st ed.). Cornell University Press. Retrieved from: https://www.cornellpress.cornell.edu/book/9781501702945/blackness-visible/.

Newton, V. A. (2022). Hypervisibility and invisibility: Black women's experiences with gendered racial microaggressions on a white campus. *Sociology of Race and Ethnicity, 9*(2), 164–178. Available at: https://doi.org/10.1177/23326492221138222.

Rajchman, J. (1995). *The identity in question*. Routledge.

Reiter, A., & Reiter, M. (2020). Microaggressions, intersectional assumptions, and the unnoticed burdens of racialized college life for Brown and Black students at a PWI. *Sociation, 19*(1), 29–44.

Wynter, S. (1994, Fall). No humans involved: An open letter to my colleagues. *Forum N.H.I.: Knowledge for the 21st Century: Knowledge on Trial, 1*(1), 42–73.

Wynter, S. (2003). Unsettling the coloniality of being/power/truth/freedom: Towards the human, after man, its overrepresentation—An argument. *CR: The New Centennial Review, 3*(3), 257–337.

Chapter 1

Blackness

Skin color is widely accepted as a noticeable marker of disparity and racial belonging. However, how we understand skin color is socially adorned, deeply sexualized, gendered, and colored. Mapedzahama and Kwansah-Aidoo (2017) underline that Blackness is not just about skin color, it is also a social construct persistently considered in opposition to whiteness. It describes whiteness and it is interiorized by it. Black scholars investigate the implication of Blackness in white settings, underlining the objectification of Black people in white spaces. They argue that Blackness is not inherent to an individual's natural color; instead, it has become a value-laden given, an object supposed to be untouched and unmediated by different contingent broad practices, past, time, and content (Mapedzahama & Kwansah-Aidoo, 2017, p. 2).

Studies on Indigenous identities in Australia underline the general prevalence, acceptance, and use of descriptors and Blackness (Mapedzahama & Kwansah-Aidoo, 2017). Historically, some scholars have freely used Black Power or Black Power Movements to designate resistance movements established by Indigenous groups organizing against colonization. Many use the description to represent the racial divide that exists between Indigenous people as the original inhabitants of the land and later colonizers (Mapedzahama & Kwansah-Aidoo, 2017).

Mapedzahama and Kwansah-Aidoo (2017) argued that the capacity of the term Blackness to meaningfully designate a group of people is questionable because Black people are not all the same and do not experience their Blackness in the same way. According to Mapedzahama and Kwansah-Aidoo, the terms Black and Blackness are highly disputed, traditionally grounded in the social construction of race, and their use, correctness, impoliteness, and significance in modern society continue to be discussed. Blackness carries with it history, depiction, culture, identity, and devoutness (Rutland, 2018). Annamma et al. (2018) raised concerns about the overrepresentation of Black, Latinx, and Native American students receiving unique education labels. These students received harsh disciplinary sanctions, were placed in the most restrictive and segregated placements, and were funneled into jails inspired by their scholarly work.

Gross-Wyrtzen (2022) defined race as a historically contingent formation and argued that Blackness emerged at different periods in North African history, taking form from Islamic expansion to the present day. It signified lesser social status and non-belonging; meanings shaped practices, discussions, and reminiscences of slavery. Garba and Sorentino (2022) stressed that the antecedence of Blackness-before-race expounds on race's rise and complexity, how race-as-reoccupation surpasses empirical decipherability, for it is the substratum via which the world is rendered intelligent. Garba and Sorentino cite Wynter's definition of race in which race measures self-assertion and sutures the modern state by assuring that "ends" are still extra-humanly set for human nature by the constraints of nature and history. Race succeeds at a high cost as a supposed form of social objectivity.

Some studies differentiate Blackness from race by outlining it as the problem latent within the generation of race. Garba and Sorentino (2022) identify Blackness as the marked distinction in the levels of sub-rationality generated within the West's classificatory system. Placing Blackness before arguing illustrates the genetic status-organizing principle of which the singularity that people have come to know as race is the expression. Garba and Sorentino stress that Blackness informs both formal and empirical approaches to accessing the axiom that regulates discernability, serving as the hermeneutical limit between orders and underscoring the leading code introducing other modes of distinction.

Race is one of the most important forms of social identity—an illustrative element of identity. It is something people see, and it is a part of individual identities that is separate from the individual's self-perception. Race matters—to an extent. Power centers have a way of dividing groups according to matters of descent, race, disability, religion, culture, and class. As C.L.R. James (1989) once wrote, race is not equal to class in colonial situations, but to see race as merely incidental is a grave error too (p. 283). Blackness is a well-marked visible identity element. It is something that people are able to see rather than something that people apply on the basis of influence.

The racial construct identity of Blackness is often used in the context of anti-Black racism as the visible "inferiority" in a white society. Banahene Adjei (2018) notes that "within visceral anti-Black racism's context, there is a hypervisibility of Blackness" (p. 3). It allows those who choose to discriminate to readily identify and assign a relative social value, a clear demarcation of social rank, status, or perceived intelligence. Tavernier (2008) couched the use of Blackness as a social stigma in the context of the Dominican Republic / Haitian prejudice and discrimination against the dark-skinned inhabitants of Hispaniola. Defined in relation to whiteness, the term "Blackness" perpetuates the negation of the "other," which becomes the basis for institutionalized anti-Black racism and the culture of imperialism. This phenomenon manifests itself in such a way that there is a stratified racism at play.

Education is a very important part of the struggle to empower disadvantaged communities. Collins (2015) describes how knowledge is the primary tool that oppressed people need in confronting discrimination and oppression. This educational knowledge helps by both offering oppressed groups knowledge about the mechanisms and processes of their oppression and, more importantly, offering them the tools to fight this oppression.

My research aligns with critical Black theorists who want Black people to embrace their Blackness, their culture, and their heritage, whatever form it takes. For instance, bell hooks (1992) warns against imitation that results in colonized people seeing themselves as they are seen in the eyes of the colonizer, which often leads racialized people to despise the very culture that was once a source of joy and spiritual fulfillment. She calls for the appropriation of this discourse as a means to embrace the tendencies that represent Blackness "one dimensionally in ways that reinforce and sustain white supremacy":

> [Black] folks who "love Blackness," that is, who have decolonized our minds and broken with the kind of white supremacist thinking that suggests we are inferior, inadequate, marked by victimization ... often find we are punished by society for daring to break with the status quo. (hooks, 1992, pp. 17–19)

However, colonial theorist Frantz Fanon (1967) criticizes the notion of embracing Blackness. For him, the Black soul as we know it is a European artifact, an existential deviation forced upon Black people by European culture. He argues that the definition of "Black" emerged from a racist culture and invariably reproduced a culture that classified humans not according to their skills and abilities but according to the color of their skin. Even though such a term might appear to be politically correct in the twenty-first century, it is still problematic. Rather than discourage racism, the expression actually perpetuates the racist stereotyping of the "other."

Emerging from the colonial discourse of Africa and other imperialist propaganda in the nineteenth century, the term "Black" has a negative connotation. Like the expressions "people of color" and "nonwhite," the term "Black" has emerged from a global cultural that has fed and continues to feed on racial discrimination and negative stereotypes that perpetuate European imperialistic ideologies and discourses.

Fanon (1967) argues that the very notion of "Blackness" itself is a construct of the societal order of oppression that was created by the oppressor. I argue that Blackness is constructed like other categories of oppression such as disability, race, gender, and sexuality. Like other social constructions, race emerges from and exists in its representation in cultural values. However, as a social construction, race is a difficult and changing concept, and we can see the implication of these constructs of marginalization on the image of non-normative bodies and minds as built through oppressive categories (Garland-Thomson, 1997). One of the interesting features of race, and Blackness in particular, is how its power is dependent upon the social acceptance of its objectivity. Of course, it may be argued—in objection to the idea of social construction—that as these categories and labeling processes are social phenomena, they are readily addressable and subject to revision. However, this view ignores the power of social construction in our contemporary culture. Human, race, and disability are themselves categories founded upon modes of social construction and signification. Indeed, it may be argued that nothing truly exists for us without some cognitive social constructions of its existence. This serves to explain why systemic discrimination is so enduring and pervasive in our culture; it is, quite simply, economical to those engaged in it.

Anti-Blackness and Anti-Black Racism

Anti-Blackness by definition means those practices, behaviors, attitudes, actions, and beliefs that marginalize, minimize, and devalue Black people. These expressions of anti-Blackness deny Black people dignity, their humanity, and often justify the overpolicing, disposability, and under- protection of Black people (Akuoko-Barfi et al., 2023; Comrie et al., 2019; Walcott, 2021; Sandhu, 2021). Similarly, anti-Black racism refers to racial prejudice directed at Black people or people who others assume to be Black (Comrie et al., 2019). This type of racism is structural and systemic (Mills, 2018). Racism alone does not capture the shade of discrimination that Black people face. It needs the prefix "anti-Black" to show which aspect of racism is being addressed.

Some of the components of anti-Black racism and anti-Blackness include destruction of identity, criminalization, health, education, and social conceptions of value. Often, Black people's identity is devalued by making them appear inferior; they are painted as uncontrolled, angry, violent, and unattractive (especially women; Comrie et al., 2019). Mwangi et al. (2018) describe the experiences of many Black campus students who say that most non-Black students fear them. Whenever many white people see them, they seem on edge. Some assume that a women will automatically turn into the stereotype of the angry Black woman. Other non-Black students avoided working with Black students on campus. These Black students expressed frustrations about these interactions because their skin color is something they have no control over (Mwangi et al., 2018). The Black students also explained that microaggressions we often experienced through the sexual fetishization of Black women or hair politics. It was like a black elephant in the room.

Black people are criminalized and overpoliced, thus leading to their overrepresentation in prison. Sharpe (2016) describes incidences in which many of her relatives were murdered by the police. In one situation, a cousin called Robert was schizophrenic. He was a university student but developed the mental health condition in his first year on campus. One day, he did not take his medication and became agitated while walking around the neighborhood. Police engaged in an eight-hour standoff at his home and shot him several times. They claimed he pointed a gun at them but it was later established that it was a toy gun. An unarmed Black man was thus shot 11 times in the back because he seemed threatening because of his height and race (Sharpe, 2016). These are the realities Black people face.

There are issues of racism and discrimination in education and health because of bigotry present in social conceptions of value, with Black people facing bigotry historically as slaves and today from the police and the rest of society. In terms of health, differential treatment of Black people in pain management testing and access to health care are forms of anti-Blackness (Comrie et al., 2019). With regard to education, Black people often fight crippling poverty and homelessness, which undermines education access. Sharpe (2014) shares the story of a twelve-year-old Black girl called Dasani who was suspended by her principle. Once that happened, she became homeless immediately. The situation is worse on campuses because higher education is essentially a white colonial space (Robinson, 2022). Anti-Blackness is evident in Canada's tertiary institution through the exclusion of Black content from the curriculum and because Black Canadians are underrepresented in leadership. Staff face workplace discrimination and there is minimal engagement around Blackness.

These spaces normalize whiteness and cultural imperialism. Cameron and Jefferies (2021) note that many Black high school students are discouraged from attending university and are instead encouraged to do vocational training. This devaluing of Black students hinders them from continuing with their education. Between 2006 and 2011, 84% of white students in Toronto graduated high school compared to 69% of Black students (Cameron & Jefferies, 2021, p. 12). These disparate outcomes are the result of the disparate and unequal treatment Black people face. Mwangi et al. (2018) add that often campus students have to contend with the lack of support from their mates from other races. For example, when Black students organize a Black Lives Matter event in university, their white friends do not participate or engage in these issues even though they are so meaningful to their friend. When these Black students then become an academic or tutor in a Canadian university, they have to deal with differential treatment from the faculty. Cameron and Jefferies (2021) stated that one Black faculty member said he had to publish 20 times more than his white colleagues to secure tenure.

This history of anti-Blackness is deep-seated. Canada's anti-Black racism largely sprang from chattel slavery that existed in its neighboring country, the United States. At the time, state-sanctioned terror reigned supreme (Joyce & Abdou, 2023). There were no voting rights and vast incarceration and separation was the reality. After abolishing slavery, some freed slaves came to Canada, but they continued to face discrimination and disenfranchisement in this new land. Now, hundreds of years later, Black people continue to be treated as unworthy (Comrie et al., 2019). The persistence of anti-immigrant sentiments against Black immigrants is an illustration of this bigotry. Even Black communities themselves have internalized this inferiority and expressed discrimination towards each other. This colorism manifests as disdain for people with darker skin tones or Afro-textured hair.

Masculinity

I was born and raised in Jamaica, where I faced myriad challenges and obstacles that inhibited my ability to succeed and survive. These challenges were compounded by the physical and emotional abuse I endured during my childhood. My father abandoned me when I was about five, and within a year of my father's leaving, my mother sent me to be raised by my grandmother. Under my grandmother's care, I received frequent beatings with various objects such as belts, sticks, and hard punches and also experienced other forms of cruelties. When I was 10, my grandmother's husband (my step-grandfather) expressed his disapproval of me living with them and asked me several times to leave their house. Because I had nowhere else to go, he took the opportunity to mentally torture me.

One Sunday afternoon, while I was at church, one of my grandmother's pastors accused me of talking to my childhood friend Junior. The pastor and my grandmother beat me so hard that my thirteen-year-old body was severely and physically damaged; the beating had a lasting impact on my adulthood. The physical and emotional abuse I endured throughout my childhood brought a lot of confusion, mistrust, and misunderstanding about the meaning of home and the meaning of parental love for a child.

Paternal abandonment and children being raised in grand-matriarchal families are not uncommon familial circumstances in Black Jamaican society. Historians and sociologists generally agree that these familial patterns are due to colonialism and the efforts of European plantation owners in colonial Jamaica to disrupt African enslaved families to ensure control of a divided workforce (Craton, 2022; Hall, 2017; Hickling, 2020; Lemonius, 2017). Males are expected to be strong, independent, and roguishly irresponsible, characteristics that make a child more vulnerable to neglect and abuse. This is how I now make sense of what happened to me.

Gender and masculinity were deeply intertwined with these interpretative frames in a colonial context, as they are intertwined with homelessness, disability, and Blackness in a Canadian context. Given the sheer extraordinary multiplicity of gender identities (as well as other interrelated dimensions of Blackness, disability, and class), to speak of not being "masculine enough" is to build on assumptions about femininity. It is important to note how Black masculine identity, a racial identity, is shown to be closely linked to heterosexuality. The significance of this is that Black homosexual activity would logically be seen as somehow a repudiation of one's identity as a Black person.

For example, in Jamaica, when men get "emotional," they are deemed disabled and too feminine, and thus, are denounced as homosexuals. This suggests that the origins of prejudice against gay men in Jamaican society may derive from the fact that they could be defined as an internal "threat to the integrity of the nuclear family" (Collins, 2004, p. 106). Moreover, as "punishment," these men suspected of a "crime" are subjected to stigmatization as deviant and predatory. The Black Jamaican community has internalized this stigmatization as an essential core of Black masculine identity itself. Chunnu (2021) notes that men in Jamaica who are suspected to be homosexuals could face "severe discrimination that often leads to violence and even death from members of the public" (p. 123). Thus, homophobia and stereotypes of Black sexuality do not function to reflect or represent reality but instead to disguise or mystify objective social relations like racism, classism, sexism, and heteronormativity. Scholars have argued that the threats present in Jamaican dancehall music may contribute to caricatures such as "batty boy must die," "bitches," "fish," "chi chi man," and "faggot" and this stigmatization of their sexuality, and particularly Black homosexuality, may be why many gay individuals in Jamaica are less authentic (Chapman & et. al, 2021; Chunnu, 2021; Edwards, 2020; Saunders, 2003). As Fassinger (2010) writes, "Their sexual identity remains hidden or undisclosed for a variety of reasons such as fear, perceived irrelevance and or being hostile" (p. 202). Thus, the challenge for Black homosexuals is that any acknowledgment—in public or in private—of their gender identity is likely to be read by their community as a rejection of its racially-based group identity. I argue that masculinity is the configuration of gender practices, which is the currently accepted answer to the problem of the legitimacy of patriarchy—the dominant position of heterosexual men (Biholar, 2022; Lewis & Carr, 2009; Thame & Thakur, 2014).

According to Collins (2004), Black political theory abstracts from matters of gender and sexuality, a salient illustration of the Black churches' resentment of homosexuality (Schalk, 2022). Black LGBT presence has been challenging to discern in public discussion and the media. Collins (2004) notes that gay Black men are forced to lead double lives, a silence and omission implicated in the rising rates of HIV/AIDs among Black people. She advocates for a more inclusive political consciousness that offers a place for diversities of eros and committed love.

Collins (2004) explored how race, class, and sex organize national social life. She makes two claims: first, she deliberates the new form of discrimination that slavery statutes and Jim Crow laws introduced. Accordingly, this strain of racism was pervasive but challenging to recognize. She made a second case for more subtle racism that remains imposed upon and internally recreated by Black communities. Collins cites numerous examples, including the ambiguous testimony of film and television. Novel forms of global capitalism frame the new racism, which disenfranchises voters and drives politics through economic influence. From this perspective, we can see how extraordinarily complex "compulsory heterosexuality" is in Jamaican society (Francis, 2021; McRuer, 2002; Milagros Early & Grundetjern, 2022; Nicolazzo, 2017; Rich, 2003). The extraordinary level of masculinity in this culture—in which even single men with no children invite "suspicion" and femininity is a by-product of service to masculine sexual power and authority—allows us to understand why many gay men in Jamaica would prefer to be "invisible," to protect themselves physically and economically. While Jamaican gay men of diverse cultural backgrounds have frequently found themselves doubly marginalized and alienated, it must be acknowledged that they have also resisted these processes of dispossession to protect their identities in flux and erasure.

It is well known that one of the most common racist stereotypes historically applied to Black men is related to their masculinity, whether in Jamaica or Canada. Black masculinity is commonly seen as a rogue agency, with Black men all too frequently represented as irresponsible "slaves" to their own body. While Jamaica has admittedly made significant strides against cultural racism, the enduring nature of this cultural myth of Black masculinity as inherently irresponsible to the point of violence remains as a testament to the cultural power of racism in Jamaican society.

Colonialism of the Mind

The normalization, indifference, acquiescence, and defeatism of the Black, Indigenous, people of color, and disabled persons are attributed to the colonialism of the mind. The colonialism of the mind refers to the subtle manifestations of the colonizers' political, economic, cultural, and religious beliefs in the victim's or the subject's mind (Fanon, 1967; Kgatla, 2018; Oelofsen, 2015). In other words, formerly colonized people internalize the attitudes of ethnic or cultural inferiority based on the feeling that the cultural values of the colonizers are inherently superior and better. There are various manifestations of colonization of the mind notable from the attitudes of Black and disabled people in the face of their historical anti-Blackness and ableism.

The colonization of the minds of Black communities was white supremacists' deliberate project to assert their dominance and obscure their white privilege. This was done by imposing on the Black communities new perspectives on life and social structure to induce them to abandon their cultural norms and adopt white norms (Kgatla, 2018, p. 149; Oelofsen, 2015, p. 135). Colonization of the mind correctly denotes that colonization does not necessarily end with the decolonization of a community in the political sense.

Therefore, the impact of the colonial project is more deeply entrenched in the subjects minds. As observed by Ngugi wa Thiongo (1983), colonial traits and ideologies are deposited in the subjects minds in various ways, including in religious doctrine and educational curricula. This is equivalent to deculturization, where the victims are pacified, controlled, and conditioned to relinquish their culture, history, and ancestral education and instead adopt Eurocentric values. This may also be equated to seasoning or brainwashing and miseducation (Kgatla, 2018, p. 148). The natural and intended consequence of the colonization of the minds of Black communities is that they have learned to feel ashamed and embarrassed of their cultural heritages and historical past. Further, Black communities have learned to accept and embrace Western culture as universal and superior. This is noted in the commonplace phenomenon in Black communities for Black people to diligently try to mirror white people, for instance, in their dressing, use of the colonizer's language, bleaching of their skin, or use of artificial hair over their own.

One of the prime examples is how missionaries functioned as key actors in the imperialism and domination by Europeans in colonized outposts. The key to both goal's sought by missionaries, conversion of Indigenous Peoples to Christianity and colonial domination, is through the fostering of an image of divinity by Western Christianity: God. Not just any God but a racialized God and thus a racialized religious ideal which creates the equation: God=Good=White. Fanon (1967) argued that "the good and merciful God cannot be black: He is a white man with bright pink cheeks" (p. 51). Thus, by implication, if divinity is "white," then having black skin made them separate from the divine and therefore inherently not good. This inherent connection between race, power, and validity had a profound impact upon the consciousness of Black people, who were indoctrinated by this white European knowledge system.

The very literature itself is also to be blamed. The oppressed and colonized Black and Indigenous peoples were exposed to European classics of civilization and taught to imitate or idolize these lives and stories. For example, we were given Shakespeare in Jamaica and told of far-off lands of which we had no inkling. The texts justify the superior and righteous nature of the European cause. Yet the oppressed, even the educated, perhaps even more the educated, imitate their conquerors from this education: in life, in style, in culture, and in manner. There is also the aspect of learned indifference, where Black communities are disinterested in fighting back against subtle manifestations of racial abuse and inequalities.

Another notable consequence of colonization of the mind is the commonplace disunity among the Black communities in their fight against racial inequalities. The colonization of the mind underscores the psychological impact of colonization, where the mentality of the colonized is eroded and colonized to the extent that the colonized internalizes the motions of racial inferiority and cultural backwardness, leading to low self-esteem and self-hate (Oelofsen, 2015, p. 138). The colonization of the mind is also relevant in the case of disabled persons. The capitalist notion or ideology of ableism has miseducated disabled persons to feel inferior and embarrassed because of their disability. Ableism is the characterization of disabled persons as inferior to non-disabled persons. This notion is problematic because it rationalizes overt and covert discrimination and social prejudice against people with disabilities.

The colonialism of the mind is also noted by various Black scholars, including Steve Biko, Frantz Fanon, Ngugi wa Thiongo, and Chinua Achebe, as an inexplicable psychological impact of colonization (Kgatla, 2018, p. 149). Biko (2019), for instance, states that owing to his Blackness, he faced the constant reality of being treated based on the racialized perception of Blackness. As such, he faced the constant reality of either fighting against the racist white gaze or internalizing the perception (Kgatla, 2018, p. 150). The inescapable conclusion from a thorough understanding of the colonization of the mind phenomenon is that decolonization of the mind is imperative if Black communities and disabled persons are to emancipate themselves and rise above the colonial entrapment of their minds. This, for instance, forms the basis of the Black Consciousness movement founded by Steve Biko in South Africa. This is best captured in Biko's statement, "Black man, you are on your own," which encourages Black people to be independent in their thinking and existence.

Fanon (1967) was the first Black theorist I read whose work made fully visible a world I had hitherto only perceived in shadows. In the post-colonial Jamaica of my youth, it was my experience that many people believed the European colonialists and empires were relics of history (Fanon, 1967). However, many others—including myself—were not so sure. To me, it seemed as though the legacy of empire endured in complex and potent ways. Indeed, when I first read Fanon—a writer I had been told was controversial for his discussion of violence and anti-colonialism—it was not his treatment of violence that resonated with me so much as his examination of the power of colonialism at the level of culture and language: a colonialism of the mind. This characteristic of "colonialism of the mind" is arguably also evident in Fanon's analysis—although implicitly rather than explicitly. Scholars have argued that colonialism continues in other forms, such as in educational institutions. It is from this perspective that my research critically explores this problem of colonialism.

There are many characteristics of colonialism, such as colonialism of the mind and the rule of (colonial) law (Adams, 1999; Césaire, 1972; Fanon, 1967). While it must be acknowledged that there exist many definitions of colonialism, it can be argued that all the definitions incorporate features such as the occupation of territories by settlers; the eradication, removal, or control of the occupants; and the exploitation of their land and resource for economic gain. However, these features do not adequately describe the full complexity of the colonial process, nor do they give us a clear understanding of why this phenomenon is so powerful and continues in modern history. Therefore, a more critically valuable approach would be to focus on the characteristics, noted by a number of scholars and commentators (Erevelles & Minear, 2010; Wynter, 2003), through which the process of colonialism operates, especially in the context of education.

Regardless of the technological or military advantage of the colonizer, such a colonial empire could not have been built or controlled without a system of indoctrination that taught the colonized peoples to accept their oppression. Through this process, colonized peoples are often mentally and ideologically subordinated to the extent that they are reduced to willing partners in their own oppression and even marginalization. Fanon (1967) argues that we are talking not only about the "racialized" body but also the "body of culture" that, in its colonial form, is assimilative and a critical tool in the subjugation of a population (p. 222). Culture is a powerful tool of hegemonic power because it controls not only how people are represented but also the very terms they can use to represent themselves.

Wynter (2003) demonstrates how European elites would periodically revise their conception of the "self" in order to reassert their claims to power in response to wider social preserves and cultural change. Thus, the concept of "race" was advanced—and quickly incorporated as a natural "given" of social order—as European society began to secularize and expand their contact with cultures outside Europe. Through this process of secularization, European culture discursively revised the "basis on which all human groups had millennially 'grounded' their descriptive statement/prescriptive statements of what it is to be human, and to reground its secularized reconception a newly projected human/subhuman distinction instead" (Wynter, 2003, p. 264).

According to Wynter (2003), the modern world is engaged in a struggle between a conception of "man" and a broader definition of "the human" in which "man" is understood to have physical, intellectual, and moral superiority. For Wynter, race is the single most effective tool of domination utilized in the modern world. The idea of race, along with other tools, supports domination by creating social identities or categories that define behaviors and relationships. Identity categorization, both on an informal and administrative level, is an everyday reality for Black disabled students. The recognition of the inequity of identifying people according to set categories has progressed from ambivalence toward anti-Black racism and other forms of marginalization to, today, an emerging acknowledgment—though still from a colonial, Eurocentric perspective—of the inherent violence of enforcing such post-colonial paradigms (Bhabha, 1994, pp. 57–68; Dei, 2022).

Césaire (1972) depicted two distinct points of view representing the world of colonialism: the point of view of the colonizers, who "throw facts at my head" and celebrate the achievements of colonization in terms of mileages of roads and railroads, and the point of view of the colonized, which focuses on the human cost of such achievements with people enslaved in the process (p. 21) This point is similarly made by Chataika et al. (2012), who noted that the roles of disability and development in postcolonialism are intertwined. Perhaps the most significant aspect of Césaire's (1972) observation is his acknowledgment of the key role of education in teaching the dominance of the colonizer's explanatory narrative: "I am talking about millions of [wo]men ... who have been taught to have an inferiority complex, to tremble, kneel, despair, and behave like flunkeys" (p. 343).

Similarly, Titchkosky (2011) notes that language is critically important in understanding representations of disability and exclusion, in that our social groups' "way of saying things" is "representative of the cultural grounds of possibility from which they emanate" (p. 74). What we say, and how we say it, not only reflects but also creates the world we live in. In other words, the exclusion is made viable and possible by how we represent excluded categorized language. It is significant how, in Titchkosky's depiction of contesting narratives, even the most absurd exclusion is rendered reasonable.

A key challenge that arises in the process of reflection upon the various topics discussed in my book is the sheer scope of this pedagogical project. Colonialism at its height encompassed the greater portion of the landmass and population of the planet and its colonization of the cultural diversity of the world continues to shape our bodies, minds, and cultural discourses to the present day. In the Jamaica of my youth, it seemed to me that we were aware—though most of us lacked the theoretical apparatus to describe it—of how colonialism left us with contradictions: politically, we claimed to have thrown off the shackles of imperial Britain, but we knew how colonialism continued to define our minds and our cultural and social practices. While the era of the European colonial empires may have passed, the colonization of the mind continued. Walter Mignolo (2012), Sylvia Wynter (2003), and Alexander Weheliye (2014) speak of this as the "coloniality of power"—something that Foucault (1994) did not take into account in his analysis of power. In this, the vestiges of colonialism remain pervasive in society. The artifacts of colonial domination are present in institutions, systems, and the structure of how we live. Nonetheless, the working of power takes its roots from colonialism, which is not just an event of the past but an ongoing productive force.

Consider the role of religion in this ongoing reproduction of power born of the colonial legacy. According to Fanon (1967), colonialism operates through a range of ideological agents, such as the church, and "dehumanizes the native, or to speak plainly, it turns him into an animal" (p. 42). Religious education through the reading of the Bible is one example of the complexity of cultural colonization in the Jamaica context. The paternalistic elements of religion and the way they permeate the politics of colonialism emboldened oppressors. In this respect, Turner (2021) argues that religion may be a legitimate justification for the most intimate and pervasive kinds of physical abuse or racial prejudices in Afro-Jamaican culture because of their deep-seated experiences of plantation slavery and colonial Christianity.

The evolution of popular religious belief in Jamaica is similar to other Caribbean islands where enslaved populations were encouraged to adopt the Christian beliefs of the European masters in that the British ruling class resisted the implications of equality associated with sharing a common faith with their enslaved population (Beckford, 2006; Cooper & Donnell, 2004; Lewin, 2017; Nettleford, 2004; Punnett & Greenidge, 2009; Picking et al., 2019). As a consequence, the enslaved African population incorporated the religious rituals and traditions of their African heritage into their everyday spiritual practices. Moreover, from the earliest manifestations of African spirituality in Jamaica, religious rituals and observations took on a political manifestation as acts of resistance against oppression and the colonial system. In the words of one commentator, these Jamaican practices represented "ritual aggression against the slave system" (Barrett & Barrett, 1997, p. 18). However, Afro-Jamaican culture is extraordinarily conflicted when it comes to religion and the Bible, for while Christianity has been co-opted and represented as a source of strength and cultural resistance to colonialism, we understand that it too is an instrument of that same colonialism.

Spirituality is both an internal belief and a mode of practice that can incorporate non-religious elements of compassion, love, ethics, and truth as much as elements more commonly classified as sacred, such as the immanent divine (the divine within us) and the transcendent divine (God, Goddess, Creator, Cosmos, etc.; Fernandes, 2003; Nicolae, 2023). Moreover, spirituality can have direct relevance to educational activism in North America. It is important to emphasize that this spirituality does not necessarily require adherence to an institutionalized belief system. For example, many feminist scholars are highly critical of the gender hierarchies and associated injustice of the systems of many organized religions (Fernandes, 2003; Ienne et al., 2017; Spencer, 2022). However, spirituality has been identified as a source of strength for many advocates for social change in the West, historically and in modern times. Fernandes (2003) states that spirituality is about social change, and it "recognizes the many differences among us yet insists on our commonalities and uses these commonalities as catalysts for transformation" (p. 59). Therefore, spirituality is a critically important issue as it cuts across political and ideological differences, with those claiming adherence to various belief systems often acting in a violent way in the view that they are engaged in a sacred practice sanctioned by their particular system.

Dei's (2002) work provocatively compels us to consider spirituality in the context of the discourse and counter-discourses of power in the world today. For example, while it may be all well and good to say that spirituality is about our individual relationship with the transcendent ... Dei leads one to reflect on why the European colonial powers focused so much attention on eradicating or suppressing the spiritual practices of colonized populations. I will argue that this explains why European colonizers devoted considerable energies to erasing or suppressing non-Western spiritual traditions whenever they could. In the context of Dei's (2002) analysis, however, perhaps the point is that this sense of our individual or even collective "powerlessness" is a consequence of the Western intellectual tradition—a sort of "learned helplessness," against which spirituality and spiritual practices fosters agency and a sense of possibility. In effect, if spiritual ritual can help us clarify and gain a greater understanding of the potential for transcendent meaning in our lives, can it be that we are empowered in a range of *other* dimensions in our daily existence? On a personal note, to be quite honest, I had never considered a connection between power and spirituality before reading Dei's argument. Of course, one cannot be ignorant of the importance of spirituality to Indigenous Peoples and even to resistance movements (from the African American Civil Rights movement based in Black churches to the importance of spirituality in Canadian First Nations protests). However, Dei seems to argue that we need to understand these not as isolated struggles but as connected in a larger context—against the "violence of Western science and colonizing knowledges" (p. 2). I feel I should also reinforce the point that Dei is not idealistic or simplistic in this analysis. For example, he writes that "it is not suggested that all local cultural knowledges are spiritual, or that religion is synonymous with spiritual" (p. 6).

Though government-run public education in the 1970s (Bourne & Owen-Wright, 2018), my experience with primary education was through missionary religious schools where the Bible was a central component of my studies. Silvera's (1992) analysis is informative as it explores the historic, political, and cultural origins of the Bible in Afro-Jamaican culture. She notes that:

> Our foreparents gained access to literacy through the Bible when they were being indoctrinated by missionaries. It provided powerful and ancient stories of strength, endurance and hope which reflected their own fight against oppression [and colonialism]. (p. 523)

Silvera's argument highlights the role of the Bible in both fuelling and shaping our understanding of the context of the Bible in Afro-Jamaican culture. Studying the Bible not only taught me literacy, a key avenue to power, but it also provided me with powerful stories of people struggling against oppression and enduring in the hope of salvation. These lessons permeate my Afro-Jamaican cultural expression, most notably in the Rastafarian beliefs (also influenced by Christianity) that infuse reggae music, for example: "I Am That I Am," (Tosh, 1977).

Rastafarianism is a significant site of convergence—in Jamaica history—of the issues of Blackness, cultural (African/hybrid) heritage, national identity, and power politics. One of the most fascinating aspects of Rastafari in Jamaican history is how it coalesced at the intersection of Jamaican spirituality, ideas of Blackness and African heritage, political resistance and social change, and popular culture.

Rastafarianism is a Messianic movement that originated in Jamaica in the 1930s but which has deep roots in the complex web of culture and politics and African spirituality that defines Jamaican religious practice. Its members believe that Ras Tafari, the great grandson of King Saheka of Shoa, who was crowned Negus of Ethiopia and took the name "Haile Selassie" (Might of the Trinity)—to which was later added the titles "King of Kings" and "Lion of the Tribe of Judah"—is the Messiah incarnated to redeem Africans exiled from the continent by white oppressors (Barrett & Barrett, 1997; Gomes, 2019; Price, 2014). The movement envisions Ethiopia as the Promised Land to which all Black people will eventually be repatriated (Barrett & Barrett, 1997, pp. 1, 81).

For me, singing this song, "I am that I am," was a mode of resistance against parental abuse, social oppression, and injustice in colonial Jamaica. Abuse from parents and others can be harsh and should be feared. Thus, there are times when I had to fight back and challenge these abuses, even if it meant that I had to jeopardize my well-being. If there were relevant laws in Jamaica, they were not observed or used to protect children from parental abuse, or other forms of abuse, at that time (Orlando, 2020).

Consequently, parents had the ultimate authority to discipline their children to the fullest extent, even if it meant abusing and seriously hurting them. Studies have found that children who commit suicide are increasingly concerned about how the normalization, at home, at church, or in the community, of parental or other people's abuse has resulted in the victims being seen as lying or problematic (Henry-Lee, 2020; Turner, 2021). The heavy burden these children have had to bear has a tremendously negative impact, not only on their young lives, but also on their adult lives and mental health.

Exploring the consistent theme of marginalization in my story allows us to see how lyrics articulate the oppression that colonization imparts upon Black bodies. This song were a form of resistance to colonization and the annihilation of the self. To illustrate the personal impact upon my own consciousness of Fanon's radical critique of colonialism and the processes of decolonization, considering this song by Peter Tosh is illuminating.

According to Brkich et al. (2012), music can be a vehicle to challenge racism and ableism or "overcome feelings of powerlessness and personal guilt" (p. 3). In the context of my youth in Jamaica, singing this song was a way to achieve an inner freedom that responds to the negativity surrounding my Blackness, masculinity, and disability. Moreover, cultural productions—most notably reggae music—remain as defining characteristics of the idealism and spirit of resistance of a Jamaica that, while often fragmented politically and racially, endeavors to sing as one in the global chorus.

Fanon's (1963) writing is particularly important to an analysis of colonization because he draws attention to the complex nature of colonialism: colonialism is not simply about conquest, domination, and economic exploitation, but more importantly, it is about mental and cultural subjugation and erasure. For Fanon, colonialism is an especially insidious and destructive process because so many of its key functions occur at mental, cultural, and pedagogical levels. Thus, unlike the wars and conquests of one European people by another—where a population retains its identity and culture—colonialism is critically concerned with cultural erasure and mental domination, resulting in a bifurcated consciousness (DuBois, 1903; Wright, 1993).

Who am I—as a Black Caribbean man who received my earliest education in a religious (European Christian) school and learned a European language (with dialect) as my native tongue? The first time I saw Shakespeare's *Othello*, I was suddenly on the outside looking at myself—but was it myself? Or was it a cultural construct of identity that had been shaped for me by colonialism? Of course, while this is a personal view, I acknowledge that I am far from alone in this regard.

Thus, colonialism was as much a pedagogical and epistemological project as it was a military, political, and economic one. It endeavored to control not only people's bodies, their social institutions, and their economic means of production and resources but also colonized populations' minds and cultures: it taught them how to see themselves through the colonizer's eyes, through the colonizer's language, just as it taught them to use the knowledge constructs and concepts of the colonizer and their conceptualization of the body.

Reconnecting to Roots

Rinaldo Walcott (2003) states that an important part of empowering Black people in Canada is reconnecting with their historical roots and culture, particularly in diaspora communities. Diaspora culture is an important expression of their heritage and identity and moves away from simplistic concepts of Blackness. One of the challenges of Black identity is that being Black has actually erased other valid identities.

Stuart Hall (2001), in defining identity as bound up with history, shows that Black people in North America are categorized simply as "Black" rather than having identity categorizations that reflect their historic heritage (p. 26). In Hall's discussion of the experiences of the Caribbean diaspora, he posits that while white people are often differentiated by their country of origin or ethnic heritage (i.e., Irish, German), Black people are identified simply as such rather than by differentiating their immensely diverse heritage. Hall describes how Black people are consistently confronted with the idea that they are always from somewhere else. In one telling episode, he describes an interview with a Caribbean man in Martinique who speaks of his African heritage in perfect "lycée" French (p. 32). This man identified as French as much as Black. This demonstrates how white people can define themselves in specific terms, such as being French, but Black people are defined racially and do not have the freedom to self-identify in other categories. Thus, studying the Black student population means grouping together people from diverse historical and social backgrounds. Some of the issues they face may be universal to all Black people, others may be specific to certain communities and economic, political, cultural, or social backgrounds.

One of the most insidious capacities of colonialism, Fanon (1963) suggests, is how Black people are taught to reject their old culture in favor of European culture, a cultural frame in which there is nothing positive to associate with being Black. He notes that Black racism is not limited to its cognitive or psychological impacts and argues that we cannot understand the complexity of racism by focusing on a single aspect of the phenomenon: "The analysis that I am undertaking is psychological. In spite of this, it is apparent to me that the effective alienation of the Black man entails an immediate recognition of social and economic realities" (p. 4). I argue that, in North America we still internalize—to a significant degree—the psychosocial representation of Black masculinity as a force that is not merely full of fear but is also imagined as inherently disruptive and threatening to the social order.

According to Fanon (1963), "Because it is a systematic negation of the other person and a furious determination to deny the other person all attributes of humanity, colonialism forces the people it dominates to ask themselves the question constantly: 'In reality, who am I?'" (p. 250). Anti-colonial theorists have long noted the important role played by the education system in ensuring the control of colonized people. Much as was the case with Indigenous children in residential schools in Canada, Black children in Euro-American colonial society were indoctrinated into a culture they had no place within: "The child was now being exposed exclusively to a culture that was a product of a world external to himself. He was being made to stand outside himself to look at himself" (Thiong'o, 1996, p. 17).

Set against this background, the analysis of the pedagogical operation of colonialism is particularly complex. Decolonization and resistance are terms that carry an immense weight of significance, for colonialism was never simply a matter of politics or economics. Its enduring legacy to the present time is cultural and psychological, for the colonialism of the mind continues to define our lives.

To use a metaphor from our computer culture, how can we decolonize when our cultural "operating system"—the collective discourses and texts we use to represent and make sense of the world around us—is built upon source code originating in nineteenth-century Western Europe and modified only by a cultural "service pack" produced by U.S. cultural industries in the twentieth century? While I am Black and have been exposed to and shaped by a range of cultures and texts over the years, my Black Caribbean cultural background remains preeminent.

However, colonialism compels me to question who I am, for I know very well how significantly this cultural background has been determined by Western European interests over the course of generations. When Fanon (1963) writes that the success of colonialism lies in how it forces the colonized to continually ask themselves, "In reality, who am I?," he is not being "defeatist"—rather, he is being a realist with regard to acknowledging the full spectrum of colonial power. This spectrum includes obvious manifestations of power—economic, racial, political, and military control—to effect domination (Wynter, 2003). In this analysis, the metaphor of the computer operating system is again useful. How can I be truly certain of a decolonized-self-status when I know that core elements of the "operating system" that I use to perceive and represent the world around me were themselves products of colonialism?

References

Adams, H. (1999). *Tortured people: The politics of colonization*. Theytus Books.

Adjei, P. B. (2018). The (em)bodiment of blackness in a visceral anti-Black racism and ableism context. *Race Ethnicity and Education, 21*(3), 275–287.

Akuoko-Barfi, C., Escobar Olivo, V., Rampersaud, M., Parada, H., & Shuster, R. (2023). "I Feel Like I Was Targeted:" Black youth navigating policing in Ontario, Canada. *Child & Youth Services*, 1–26.

Annamma, S. A., Ferri, B. A., & Connor, D. J. (2018). Disability critical race theory: Exploring the intersectional lineage, emergence, and potential futures of DisCrit in education. *Review of Research in Education, 42*(1), 46–71. https://doi.org/10.3102/0091732x18759041.

Barrett, L., & Barrett, L. E. (1997). *The rastafarians*. Beacon Press.

Beckford, R. (2006). *Jesus dub: Theology, music and social change*. Routledge.

Bhabha, H. K. (1994). *The location of culture*. Routledge.

Biholar, R. (2022). Discriminatory Laws: The normalisation of sexual violence in anglophone Caribbean sexual violence laws. In *Critical Caribbean Perspectives on Preventing Gender-Based Violence* (pp. 44–64). Routledge.

Bourne, P. A., & Owen-Wright, R. (2018). Education in Jamaica: A need for redefinition and a changing of the old philosophy of education. *International Journal of Research in Humanities and Social Studies, 5*(2), 36–41.

Biko, S. (2019). Black Consciousness and the quest for a true humanity. In *Toward a Just World Order* (pp. 25–33). Routledge.

Brkich, C. A., McBride, H., & Flagg, L. (2012). Music as a weapon: Using popular culture to combat social injustice. *The Georgia Social Studies Journal, 2*(1), 1–9.

Césaire, A. (1972). *Discourse on colonialism*. Trans. J. Pinkham. Monthly Review Press.

Chapman, N., Maharaj, S., Seeberan, M., & Houlder, E. (2021). Heterosexism and homophobia in the Caribbean dancehall context. *The Thinker, 89*(4), 38–44.

Chataika, T., Mckenzie, J. A., Swart, E., & Lyner-Cleophas, M. (2012). Access to education in Africa: Responding to the United Nations convention on the rights of persons with disabilities. *Disability & Society, 27*(3), 385–398.

Chunnu, W. M. (2021). Battyboy must die! Dancehall, class and religion in Jamaican homophobia. *European Journal of Cultural Studies, 24*(1), 123–142.

Collins, P. H. (2004). Prisons for our bodies, closets for our minds: Racism, heterosexism and Black sexuality. In *Black sexual politics, African Americans, gender and the new racism* (pp. 87–116). Routledge.

Collins, P. H. (2015). Intersectionality's definitional dilemmas. *Annual Review of Sociology, 41*, 1–20. Retrieved from https://journals-scholarsportal-info.myaccess.library.utoronto.ca/pdf/03600572/v41inone/1_idd.xml.

Cooper, C., & Donnell, A. (2004). Jamaican popular culture: Introduction. *Interventions, 6*(1), 1–17.

Comrie, J. W., Landor, A. M., Riley, K. T., & Williamson, J. D. (2019). Anti-blackness/colorism. *Moving Toward Antibigotry, 74*, 1–8.

Cameron, E. S., & Jefferies, K. (2021). Anti-Black racism in Canadian education: A call to action to support the next generation. *Healthy Populations Journal, 1*(1), 11–16. https://doi.org/10.15273/hpj.v1i1.10587.

Craton, M. (2022). The passion to exist: Slave rebellions in the British West Indies, 1650–1832. In *The Atlantic Slave Trade* (pp. 259–278). Routledge.

Dei, G. J. S. (2002). Spiritual knowing and transformative learning. In *Expanding the boundaries of transformative learning: Essays on theory and praxis* (pp. 121–133). New York: Palgrave Macmillan US.

Dei, G. J. S. (2022). Cosmopolitanism or multiculturalism? Towards an anti-Colonial Reading. *International Journal for Talent Development and Creativity, 10*(1), 31–44.

Du Bois, W. E. B. (1903). *The souls of black folk*. A.C. McClurg & Co.

Edwards, S. R. (2020). *Murder Music: A content analysis of anti-LGBT Lyrics in Jamaican dancehall songs*. Western Illinois University.

Erevelles, N., & Minear, A. (2010). Unspeakable offences: Untangling race and disability in discourses of intersectionality. *Journal of Literary Cultural & Disability Studies, 4*(2), 127–146.

Fanon, F. (1963). *The wretched of the earth*. Grove Press.

Fanon, F. (1967). *Black skin, white masks*. Trans. Charles Lam Markmann. Grove Press.

Fassinger, R. E. et al. (2010). *Towards an Affirmative Lesbian, Gay, Bisexual and Transgender Leadership Paradigm. American Psychologist, 65*(3), 201–215.

Fernandes, L. (2003). *Transforming feminist practice: Non-violence, social justice, and the possibilities of a spiritualized feminism*. San Francisco, CA: Aunt Lute Books.

Foucault, M. (1994). Subjectivity and truth. In J. Faubion (Ed.), *Ethics: Subjectivity and truth* (pp. 87–92). New Press.

Francis, D. A. (2021). "A gay agenda": Troubling compulsory heterosexuality in a South African university classroom. *Teaching Sociology, 49*(3), 278–290.

Garba, T. P., & Sorentino, S.-M. (2022). Blackness before race and race as reoccupation: Reading Sylvia Wynter with Hans Blumenberg. *Political Theology*, 1–22. https://doi.org/10.1080/1462317x.2022.2079216.

Garland-Thomson, R. (1997). *Extraordinary bodies: Figuring physical disability in American culture and literature*. Columbia University Press.

Gomes, S. (2019). Global sufferahs: Rastafari cosmopolitan citizenship. *Tout Moun Caribbean Journal of Cultural Studies, 5*(1).

Gross-Wyrtzen, L. (2022). 'There is no race here': On blackness, slavery, and disavowal in North Africa and North African studies. *The Journal of North African Studies, 28*(3), 635–665. https://doi.org/10.1080/13629387.2022.2089124.

Hall, S. (2001). Negotiating Caribbean identities. In B. Meeks & F. Lindahl (Eds.), *New Caribbean thought: A reader* (pp. 24–39). University of the West Indies Press.

Hall, S. (2017). *Familiar stranger: A life between two islands*. Duke University Press.

Henry-Lee, A. (2020). Children in violent circumstances. In *Endangered and transformative childhood in Caribbean Small Island Developing States* (pp. 103–140). Palgrave Macmillan. https://doi.org/10.1007/978-3-030-25568-8_5.

Hickling, F. W. (2020). Owning our madness: Contributions of Jamaican psychiatry to decolonizing global mental health. *Transcultural Psychiatry, 57*(1), 19–31.

hooks, b. (1992). *Black looks: Race and representation.* South End Press.

Ienne, A., Fernandes, R. A. Q., & Puggina, A. C. (2017). Does the spirituality of nurses interfere in the record of spiritual suffering diagnosis?. *Escola Anna Nery, 22.*

James, C. L. R. (1989). *The Black Jacobins—Toussaint l'Ouverture & the San Domingo Revolution.* Vintage Books.

Joyce, S. & Abdou, E. (2023). Dismantling curricular statues: Critically examining anti-Black racism in representations of Ancient Africa in Canadian textbooks. *Canadian Journal of Education / Revue canadienne de l'éducation, 46*(4), 1051–1082. https://doi.org/10.53967/cje-rce.5793.

Kgatla, S. (2018). The decolonisation of the mind. Black consciousness community projects by the Limpopo Council of Churches. *Missionalia, 46,* 146–162. Available at: https://doi.org/10.7832/46-1-270.

Lemonius, M. (2017). "Deviously ingenious": British colonialism in Jamaica. *Peace Research,* 79–103.

Lewin, O. (2017). Jamaica. In *the Garland Encyclopedia of World Music* (pp. 896–913). Routledge.

Lewis, A., & Carr, R. (2009). *Gender, Sexuality, Identity, and exclusion: Sketching the outlines of the Jamaican popular nationalist project.*

Mapedzahama, V., & Kwansah-Aidoo, K. (2017). Blackness as burden? The lived experience of black Africans in Australia. *Sage Open, 7*(3). http://journals.sagepub.com/doi/pdf/10.1177/2158244017720483.

McRuer, R. (2002). Compulsory able-bodiness and queer/disabled existence. In L. Davis (Ed.), *Disability studies reader* (2nd ed., pp. 301–308). Routledge.

Mignolo, W. D. (2012). *Local histories/global designs: Coloniality, subaltern knowledges, and border thinking.* Princeton University Press.

Milagros Early, A., & Grundetjern, H. (2022). The role of sex and compulsory heterosexuality within the rural methamphetamine market. *Crime & Delinquency, 70*(6–7). https://doi.org/10.1177/00111287221077644.

Mills, C. W. (2018). *Blackness visible: Essays on philosophy and race.* Cornell University Press.

Mwangi, G., Thelamour, B., Ijeoma, E., & Carpenter, A. (2018). "Black elephant in the room": Black students contextualizing campus racial climate within U.S. racial climate. *Journal of College Student Development, 59*(4), 456–474. https://doi.org/10.1353/csd.2018.0042.

Nettleford, R. (2004). Migration, transmission and maintenance of the intangible heritage. *Museum International, 56*(1–2), 78–83.

Nicolae, T. (2023). The western revival of goddess worship. *Feminist Theology, 31*(2), 130–142.

Nicolazzo, Z. (2017). Compulsory heterogenderism: A collective case study. *NASPA Journal About Women in Higher Education*, 10(3), 245–261.

Oelofsen, R. (2015). Decolonisation of the African mind and intellectual landscape. *Phronimon*, 1616(2), 130–146.

Orlando, L. E. A. (2020). *Culturally sensitive parenting counseling, corporal punishment, and early childhood development in Grenada* [Unpublished doctoral dissertation]. Walden University.

Picking, D., Delgoda, R., & Vandebroek, I. (2019). Traditional knowledge systems and the role of traditional medicine in Jamaica. *CABI Reviews* (2019), 1–13.

Price, C. (2014). The cultural production of a black messiah: Ethiopianism and the rastafari. *Journal of Africana Religions*, 2(3), 418–433.

Punnett, B. J., & Greenidge, D. (2009). *Cultural mythology and global leadership in the Caribbean islands* (pp. 65–78). Cheltenham: Edward Elgar Publishing.

Rich, A. C. (2003). Compulsory heterosexuality and lesbian existence (1980). *Journal of Women's History*, 15(3), 11–48.

Robinson, O. (2022). Black affirming pedagogy: Reflections on the premises, challenges and possibilities of mainstreaming antiracist black pedagogy in Canadian sociology. *Canadian Review of Sociology/Revue canadienne de sociologie*, 59(4), 451–469. https://doi.org/10.1111/cars.12400.

Rutland, T. (2018). *Displacing blackness: Planning, power, and race in twentieth-century Halifax*. University of Toronto Press.

Sandhu, D. (2021). A reasonable alternative to guilt: Flight and anti-Black racism. *Windsor Rev. Legal & Soc. Issues*, 42, 51.

Saunders, P. (2003). *Is not everything good to eat, good to talk*: Sexual economy and dancehall music in the global marketplace. *Small Axe*, 13, 95–115.

Schalk, S. (2022). *Black disability politics* (p. 219). Duke University Press.

Sharpe, C. (2014). Black studies: In the Wake. *The Black Scholar*, 44(2), 59-69. Retrieved from http://www.jstor.org/stable/10.5816/blackscholar.44.2.0059.

Sharpe, C. (2016). *In the wake: On blackness and being*. Duke University Press.

Silvera, M. (1992). Man royals and sodomites: Some thoughts on the invisibility of Afro-Caribbean lesbians. *Feminist Studies*, 1 8(3), 521–532.

Spencer, A. M. (2022). The rise of an eco-spiritual imaginary: Ecology and spirituality as decolonial protest in contemporary multi-ethnic American literature.

Tavernier, L.A. (2008). The stigma of blackness: Anti-Haitianism in the Dominican Republic. *Socialism and Democracy*, 22(3), 96–104.

Thame, M., & Thakur, D. (2014). *Patriarchal state and the development of gender policy in Jamaica*.

Thiong'o, N. W. (1996). *Decolonising the mind: The politics of language in African literature*. Heinemann.

Titchkosky, T. (2011). *The question of access: Disability, space, meaning*. University of Toronto Press.

Tosh, P. (1977). I am that I am [Song]. On *Equal Rights*. Columbia Records. Retrieved from https://songmeanings.com/songs/view/3530822107858480209/.

Turner, C. (2021). Conceal to reveal: Reflections on sexual violence and theological discourses in the African Caribbean. In J. R. Reaves, D. Tombs, & R. Alvear (Eds.), *When did we see you naked?: Jesus as a victim of sexual abuse* (chap. 8). SCM Press.

Walcott, R. (2003). *Black like who? Writing Black Canada*. Insomniac Press.

Walcott, R. (2021). *On property: Policing, prisons, and the call for abolition* (Vol. 2). Biblioasis.

Wa Thiong'o, N. (1983). Education for a national culture. *Barrel of a Pen: Resistance to Repression in Neo-Colonial Kenya*. Trenton, NJ: Africa of the World P, 100.

Weheliye, A. G. (2014). *Habeas viscus: Racializing assemblages, biopolitics, and black feminist theories of the human*. Duke University Press.

Wright, R. (1993). *Native son: And how bigger was born*. Harper Perennial Press.

Wynter, S. (2003). Unsettling the coloniality of being/power/truth/freedom: Towards the human, after man, its overrepresentation—An argument. *CR: The New Centennial Review, 3*(3), 257–337.

Chapter 2

Disability

From a very young age, I was strongly attracted to schooling. Unfortunately, my school was a three-mile walk from my grandmother's home, and each day, I had to walk to and from school under the scourging tropical sun or soaking rain. Although education was important to me, I could not afford to attend school on a regular basis, and my grandmother raised a punitive hand rather than a helping hand to facilitate my efforts.

Compounding these circumstances, although I loved the idea of learning and listening to my teachers, the words they wrote on the board, or that were in the books we read, often did not make sense to me. However, despite this situation, I never gave up hope of pursuing my goals in life.

In addition to the physical and emotional abuse, I faced a new problem—severe financial difficulties that made it impossible for me to pursue my education independently. After my grandmother's husband lost his job, my grandmother informed me that my father was not supporting me and she could not afford to send me to school. Unfortunately, I had to collect and sell soft drink bottles and coconuts to make a few dollars. While this enabled me to continue attending school, as my grades dropped and other students continued to ridicule me inside and outside the classroom, I developed an inferiority complex.

I realized then, unquestioningly, that I was "broken"—a personal observation that did not go unnoticed by my fellow students and family. My grandmother was embarrassed to have a broken grandson. With my mother's assistance, one day my grandmother decided to punish me for not being "man enough" by tying me to a post on the veranda of the house and beating me until I lost consciousness. These beatings left visible scars on my body, and even though my teachers questioned my grandmother about them, the abuse continued. To compound my abuse, I was also called derogatory names, teased, and humiliated in public by the other students and people in the community. Consequently, I dropped out of high school when I was 14 years old, and by the age of 15, I wandered the streets of my town as a young homeless boy and high school drop-out.

It is important to emphasize that neither my grandmother nor mother, nor even myself, saw my learning difficulties as an instance of disability. Rather, it was framed within the cultural context of Jamaican society, which privileged the cultural production of masculinity. My grandmother saw me, and indeed I saw myself at the time, as a broken man and abandoned me as being without value. While this was certainly incredibly hard to live through, fortunately, after years of struggle, education, research, and inquiry into disability, Blackness, and cultural studies, I have come to understand how intersectionality renders our interpretation and experience of disability challenging and complex.

Alongside Blackness, disability is another identity category that serves to define and delineate social cohesion and patterns of dominance. According to the World Health Organization (WHO, 2023), around the world, people with disabilities face many inequities, such as unfair treatment, stigma, discrimination, poverty, exclusion from education and employment, and barriers within the health care system itself. Given the "rate" of disability in any population (see World Report on Disability, 2011), all of us are connected to disability, if not personally, then through family and friends. Furthermore, because there is a strong likelihood that as we age, we will encounter vision loss, such as macular degeneration, or mobility impairments of one sort or another, disability is something we will nearly all share eventually.

Whether we realize it or not, everyone is a member of the disability community directly or indirectly. As disability is something that unites us all, the study of disability—as a sense-making device and a multifaceted construct, including a range of constituent discursive practices—is of critical value to the human collective. In Western culture, disability is often represented in terms of a narrative of tragedy; it is projected as a tragic loss that removes or alienates the individual from the general population (Anand, 2020; Berger & Wilbers, 2021; Davis, 2013; Goodley, 2013; Michalko, 2002). In contrast, I am interested in the narrative of daily university experience and seek a better understanding of how disability is a fact of life for so many of us. Narratives that illuminate the incorporation of Blackness and disability into daily existence as an everyday reality are something that I find fascinating. For me, these stories are about the endless adaptability of human beings and the sheer diversity of human experience.

In this critical analysis, the human body is a site of enduring contestations of power in our society, and we must more clearly understand the processes of inscription and reading—the rules of engagement in this public arena—if we are to foster greater equity and humanity in our interactions with our fellow beings. My, and my grandmother's, interpretation of my brokenness was part of a culturally framed interpretation that served the interests of colonial power and has inscribed generations of Afro-Jamaican bodies in complex ways.

Internalizing my disability was rendered all the more complex by the requirement of the performance of (Afro-Jamaican) masculinity in Jamaican society. As Alcoff (1999) suggests, "Racism and colonialism create significant challenges for the creation of equilibrium in one's body image" (p. 18). This suggestion explains, at least in part, why the appearance of disability in my personal experience did not immediately strike me as an instance of disability. It was only through years of struggle to educate myself that I was able to more critically engage with this experience and achieve some measure of "equilibrium" in my body image, recognizing the discursive inscriptions of colonialism on my body and masculinity and the possibility of performative disruption of these discourses.

Disability represents a critical platform for resistance to our social institutions' tendency to define "normal" status. Moreover, the concept of "disability" itself has deep cultural roots in Euro-American society as an imprecise and sometimes flawed discriminatory label (Davis, 1995; Goodley, 2014; Garland-Thomson, 2020; Michalko, 2009). In this light, for the concept of "disability" to be effective in an educational context, it must be revisited from a range of critical perspectives to interrogate the concept and construction of "normality," thereby fostering a more egalitarian opposite to the social order.

Post-Traumatic Stress Disorder

This story lies in a personal experience of the learning disability assessment test at the University of Toronto. During my first-year undergraduate studies, one of my instructors, noticing that I took longer than the scheduled time to complete my exams, recommended that I go to the university's Accessibility Services office for a learning assessment. Two days after a lengthy six-hour test, a psychoeducational consultant informed me that I have a learning disability. About 20 racialized students I know were also assessed at that time, and the vast majority—approximately 90%—were also assessed as having a learning disability.

These are the tests that I was later requested to retake at the start of my PhD journey. My academic accessibility advisor informed me that I had to renew my accommodations with the Accessibility Services office. She also told me that my accommodation file must be updated in order to continue to receive accommodation. This was shocking to me because I received accommodations throughout my undergraduate and master's degree studies at the same university and through the same office. She recommended that I present myself for another assessment test. After a series of tests, lasting eight days and consisting of 15 and a half hours of testing with two different psychologists, one of the psychologists diagnosed me with post-traumatic stress disorder (PTSD), for which she said the only cure was treatment with medication. I felt intimidated, nervous, fearful, and anxious throughout the administration of the various tests.

As a graduate student studying for a PhD, this was disconcerting and stressful and contributed to feelings of trauma. This trauma emerged because of the stigma that is attached to being Black and having a learning disability in a graduate studies program. I experienced an extraordinary fear because of this diagnosis, and I was concerned about what this diagnosis would mean to me, including a concern for how my peers and mentors would view me in the program. Stigma is a scary experience and when it is attached to Blackness and a learning disability, it can contribute to questioning one's ability. Again, I was left to ask, "Who am I?"

This experience took me through a range of emotional responses that I have yet to fully resolve. While I have extensive experience with disability in theory and practice, being labeled with PTSD, necessitating ongoing medication to maintain a normative state, left me somewhat confused. My emotional responses wrestled with my critical understanding of issues related to this diagnosis. I struggled personally with the issues of labeling and stigma, normality and deviance, the performance of normality (with the assistance of medication), and general expectations of the desirability of the normative condition (Williams et al., 2022).

Coincidentally, this personal experience occurred during a period in which PTSD has become a prominent story in the Canadian news media. The news articles were of particular concern because they revealed the stigmatization that linked PTSD to deviant behaviors, such as substance abuse and crimes of violence, but also the role of "experts" defining PTSD in ways that augmented their authority while sensationalizing the condition with dramatic statistics (Engel & Logan, 2013; Johanssen & Garrisi, 2020).

While it must be emphasized that there is nothing wrong with having a learning disability or PTSD, the history of these concepts—particularly in terms of labeling, segregation, and differential treatment in the field of education—can cause concern to any individual (such as myself) who has been designated thus. Given my personal perspective on equity as someone with a Black Caribbean background, the issues of power and discrimination that have historically been associated with the assessment of disability are unsettling.

The phenomenon of PTSD has long been recognized, even if it has only recently come to be formally incorporated into the language of medicine. For instance, during the American Civil War, PTSD was conceptualized as "soldier's heart" (Schroeder-Lein, 2015), the symptoms of which were "palpitations, rapid heartbeat, and lightheadedness ... related to severe mental or emotional stress" (p. 128). PTSD has doubtlessly existed in every war; however, opinion has varied about whether PTSD is a deficiency of the PTSD sufferer or a by-product of a pathogenic environment. As Withuis (2008) writes of the First World War, "Soldiers who today would be defined as ill were executed as deserters" (p. 9).

Although PTSD has become an accepted disorder, recognized by both scholars and policymakers, there continues to be some controversy over the political functions of PTSD. Bloche (2011) writes that PTSD has attracted numerous skeptics who believe that PTSD is a failure of "courage and resilience" that prevents the people said to have it "from taking responsibility for their own lives" (p. 68).

As the above discussion indicates, there is considerable reason to be concerned about being assessed as possessing a disability. First, it is necessary to recognize that while such assessments are often arbitrary, they nonetheless produce considerable cultural meaning that has historically been applied in a discriminatory fashion. Second, it must be acknowledged that this discriminatory process has—in its implied construction of a "normality" or standard of normalcy—clear analogues to discriminatory practices that have historically reinforced sex, race, and gender discrimination. This discrimination gains acceptance through a framework according to which only certain types of people are considered full social participants. Discrimination then takes a shape that is similar to that of colonial oppression.

Once it is acknowledged that PTSD is not the victim's fault and that it is a disability in the ways it renders people unable to function properly in ordinary life, then there are important political repercussions. The first such repercussion is that the victim is not responsible for the disability. The responsibility shifts to the state or to other individuals (such as abusive spouses). However, if the divisions between these zones are not so sharp—if, in fact, a home or a neighborhood can function in the same way as a war zone—then it becomes more difficult to classify PTSD as a disability. As long as PTSD sufferers are actually in circumstances of genuine threat, they cannot be said to be disabled; rather, their PTSD symptoms will make them more likely to take the kinds of actions that will assist in their survival (Carter et al., 2020; Roberson & Carter, 2022; Schroeder-Lein, 2015; Williams et al., 2018). It then becomes plausible for the disability of PTSD to give rise to civic and criminal penalties, or in the case of warfare, it can be treated therapeutically by the state on whose behalf individuals acquire PTSD in the first place.

PTSD presents a useful opportunity for addressing a number of questions related to disability, in particular the question of what society needs disability to be. For some people, the very existence of PTSD as a recognized disability presents a challenge to the symbolic integrity and strength of a society, especially as such strength is symbolized by the military. For some, PTSD is an indicator of personal moral or character failings. For others, PTSD is a disability that calls attention, not to a deficiency of those who suffer from it, but to the violence that characterizes so much of human life, from the battlefield to the bedroom (Bauman, 2013).

One way of understanding the underlying politics of the definition and treatment of PTSD is through the notion of zones, which are themselves cultural constructs. In this critical analysis, "zones" are defined as socially constructed areas of activity in which subjects participate; a zone is something like a context. In looking at education, zones would be such areas of activity as the classroom, extracurriculars, and Accessibility Services, as well as processes such as testing.

Consider, for example, the American Psychological Association's (2000) diagnostic criteria for PTSD, which include the following criterion: "The disturbance causes clinically significant distress or impairment in social, occupational, or other important areas of functioning" (p. 256). As Chemtob et al. (1988) pointed out in their seminal definition of PTSD, some of the characteristics of this disorder—including hypervigilance and rapid response to perceived threats—are highly useful in actual combat situations. The imagined biological basis for this aspect of PTSD is the so-called fight or flight response, which employs adrenaline and other neurochemical control mechanisms to generate hypervigilance and other forms of response to real and perceived threats (Everly & Lating, 2013).

In terms of the theory of zones noted previously, PTSD—as supposed in the scientific discourse—appears to have replaced a premodern understanding of zones of masculinity versus zones of cowardice and reconfigured them as zones of combat versus zones of non-combat. The "scientific understanding" of PTSD made it easier to shift the essence of this disability from the zone of judgmental gender expectation to the zone of an assessment. If PTSD is reconfigured as a "disorder" that arises from some kind of faulty zone within society (such as zones of war, domestic abuse, or crime), then the treatment of PTSD necessarily involves removing sufferers from such zones and rehabilitating them in a zone of normalcy; the disabled person, abused spouse, or child rape victim must be brought back home, literally and therapeutically.

Consequently, examining the nature, characteristics, and evolution of different approaches to PTSD offers an opportunity to understand what various segments of Canadian society require PTSD-related disability to be and for what reasons. Clearly, the definition of PTSD-related disability and its consequent treatment reflect irreconcilable political viewpoints. Here, the definition and treatment of PTSD as a disability can be understood not only scientifically but also as the end result of a process of political contestation between various parties. In other words, any attempt to define PTSD solely as a biological phenomenon fails. While PTSD is certainly associated with a physiological substrate of detectable symptoms (Agaibi & Wilson, 2005; Cohen et al., 2009), these symptoms can only be labeled as a disability within the context of a cultural zone.

Having provided an indication of how the definition of PTSD as a disability is reliant on the cultural factors of distinct zones, it is possible to apply this theory to real-world cases of PTSD definition, treatment, and lack of treatment to reach relevant conclusions about what Canadian and other societies need PTSD-related disability to be and why. Clegg et al. (2006) wrote that there are three kinds of power, namely formal, informal, and hidden power. Hidden power was described as follows:

> It does not focus just on observable behavior but seeks to make an interpretive understanding of the intentions that are seen to lie behind social actions .... These come into play, especially, when choices are made concerning what agenda items are ruled in or ruled out; when it is determined that, strategically, for whatever reasons, some areas remain a zone of non-decision rather than decision. (p. 210)

A historical overview of PTSD indicates that the clarification must have first arisen in formal combat situations, in which the fighters were more likely to be men (Schroeder, 2008). Given the machismo of warfare, it is in the interest of all militarist societies to pretend that warfare is noble and that warriors are somehow supermen. Soldiers with PTSD returning from the Civil War were disabled in the sense that their hypervigilance and other PTSD symptoms actively prevented them from being able to live ordinary lives as farmers, businesspeople, fathers, or spouses. On the other hand, a woman with PTSD who lives with an actively abusive husband is not necessarily disabled by her PTSD because her condition might be responsible for increasing her chances of survival. Thus, even though it is possible to reach a consensus that PTSD is a genuine disorder, it is far more difficult—indeed impossible—to reach an objective consensus on whether PTSD is a disability. Perhaps such consensus is even not desirable. Whether PTSD counts as a disability depends on the distinctions between zones (such as zones of war versus zones of "peaceful" domestic life, as well as zones of masculinity versus cowardice) and how cultures make sense of such zones.

To name PTSD is already to acknowledge that warfare brings about collateral damage on all sides and that warriors are subject to the same pains, traumas, and disabilities as anyone else. When modern medical methods and scientific research made it difficult to continue ignoring PTSD, attempts were made to redefine it as a personal limitation rather than an indictment of violence in society. At this stage in the evolution of PTSD discourse, PTSD was either stated or hinted to be cowardice, weakness, or, at any rate, some kind of deficiency on the part of the sufferer. PTSD is classified more as a personal pathology (for which responsibility shifts to the sufferer) than a disease (for which responsibility shifts to the system in which the disease arises). Gender expectations blamed individuals, particularly men, for not living up to what society demanded of them.

Two critical readings had particular resonance for me in reflecting upon the PTSD diagnosis. Titchkosky (2000), in exploring the role of the "official text producers" of a society in terms of defining disability, observed:

> Such official definers of disability have usually come from medical jurisdictions, but sociologists, too, have a long history of producing textual knowledge on and about disabled people. The latter has typically treated disabled people as expressions of the problem of involuntary deviance, subject to processes of stigmatization who employ a variety of techniques and technologies in order to manage, cope with, or hide the problems that impaired senses, minds and/or bodies are assumed to generate. (pp. 198–199)

This observation has clear relevance to both my personal experience with a medical diagnosis of disability and PTSD and to news articles on PTSD and stigmatization. "However [wo]men define something as real, it will be real in its consequences" (Thomas, 1971, p. 274). Similarly, Titchkosky (2007) notes that there are "real consequences for the ways in which disability [and Blackness] can be read, written, thought about, lived" (p. 12). Hanisch (2006) argues that the "official text producers" in the period of second wave feminism believed that women's discontent with their social condition was—in the view of the medical establishment—a medical/psychological condition that could be "cured" with therapy:

> Therapy assumes that someone is sick and that there is a cure, e.g., a personal solution. I am greatly offended that I or any other woman is thought to need therapy in the first place. Women are messed over, not messed up! (p. 2)

Consider, as well, Taylor's (2011) indication of how the medical model of disability—which views disability as a medical condition (e.g., visual impairment, mobility impairment), a view that is surprisingly resilient even to the present day—identifies people with disabilities as being determined by their bodies. She notes that "the medical model of disability positioned the disabled body as working incorrectly, as being unhealthy and abnormal, as in need of a cure" (p. 194).

The success of oppressive forces in our society lies in their capacity to stigmatize us within the frame of a defined identity. Consider, for example, how in news articles, PTSD is closely associated with deviant behaviors (domestic violence, drug abuse, addiction, suicide). The stigma of PTSD is then attached to these problems, thereby attaching our own identity to them. The stigma extends beyond the element of PTSD and to factors only related to it statistically.

Problem People

The marginality that disabled students have experienced in the university environment is evident in the way they are presumed to be problems or trouble to be dealt with. Michalko's (2009) discussion of disability shows how disability has become an element of culture that is perceived to be trouble. Thus, disabled people are people who have problems to be dealt with.

This normalization of the disabled as a problem group has led to the idea that disability must be eliminated from the social order, or failing that, hidden or mitigated. Michalko (2009) points out that disability is normalized in such a way that people have learned to not engage with the disability of another person. He adds that disability is a social element that gives evidence of how people understand the norming of what their disability may be and how other people experience disability.

Since disability is an element of identity that is outside the self, and it is something that people may not always see, it is important to understand how it is that identity is negotiated and how the experience of living with disability changes from one social setting to the next. Low (1996) investigated the issue of disability on a college campus to understand how the students negotiate the process of being disabled in some contexts but able-bodied in others. The researcher concluded that a contradiction exists when an individual has to negotiate the nature of their disability. Given this contradiction, the student can face difficulties related to their expectations of accommodation and how the appetite for these accommodations depend on their environment. My learning disability was "invisible" to my grandmother, my mother, other students, and the community. Accordingly, I was punished and abandoned because my puzzlingly broken body was symbolic of a deprivation of hope or possibility.

While it is common to assume that "disability" is in some bodies and not in others, disability scholars have argued that it is, in fact, in the social spaces between bodies (McGuire, 2010, p. 2; see also Michalko, 2002; Titchkosky, 2007). "Brokenness" is, then, not in individual bodies; it is enacted between people. Within this context, critical disability scholars suggest that the conceptualization of disability as "brokenness" is related to taken-for-granted conceptions of a loss of hope and possibility. In this sense, "hope and, with it, possibility, therefore become tied to non-disability ... [impairment] is conceived of as a life without possibility" (McGuire, 2010, p. 6; see also Titchkosky, 2005).

For instance, "Disability is [commonly] understood and experienced ... as a disturbance to the 'normal' biology of the body. It is conceived of not as a collective matter, but as an individual one" (Michalko, 2009, p. 101; see also Levinas, 1969). As Arendt (1958) observes, while bodies have undeniable physicality, they also exist in the meanings ascribed to them in social spaces between individuals: "In acting and speaking, [wo]men show who they are, reveal actively their unique personal identities ... while their physical identities appear without any activity of their own in the unique shape of the body and sound of voice" (p. 179). For me, this quotation regarding how we reveal our identities to others has clear relevance to the concept of embodiment and "all the many and various ways that we (self and other) accomplish relations to being in possession of the bodies that we are" (Titchkosky, 2007, p. 13).

One of the most significant aspects of the theory of embodiment and its relation to meaning making is the potential for disruptive readings; that is, the capacity to "disrupt the taken-for-granted relations of embodiment" (Titchkosky, 2007, p. 13). My concern for the body problem raised by Arendt is informed in part by my personal experience growing up in Jamaica—where I was read, categorized, and defined by others on the basis of Blackness and disability.

Growing up, I believed that people's view of me was shaped by the social, economic, and political conditions of our environment and not necessarily by any particular performance of my own. It sometimes seemed like I was a tabula rasa, or blank slate, upon which people—often members of my own family—projected a range of preconceptions about Blackness, masculinity, and disability. My grandmother often commented about my physical appearance that "anything Black is not good." She went on to tell me that I was worthless and ineffective and that I would never achieve anything good in my life. They also told me to "man up" and act like a "real man." It was a very emotional, humiliating, and dehumanizing experience to endure. Arendt (1958) suggests that we make our physical identity "appear" to others through our actions but not necessarily with explicit consciousness of doing so. In contrast, the concept of embodiment suggests an active, performative aspect. In other words, Arendt suggests we enact our embodiment with some possibility of conscious intentionality. But can this be said for all of us?

Consider the problem of students with disabilities. One of my research interests in the field of disability studies is the dynamic relationship that has historically existed between students with disabilities and educational institutions. It is fascinating to see how students with disabilities have historically been inscribed by educational institutions in ways analogous to how in my youth I found myself serving as a tabula rasa for others in Jamaica.

For example, children with disabilities are not active agents or actors to the same degree as adults with disabilities. Because their psychological and cognitive development has not matured, some people argue that children cannot enact their embodiment as we adults can. Indeed, their immaturity renders them acutely vulnerable to having their identities inscribed by external forces with limited input or influence from them. This being said, we can see how Arendt's (1958) conception of the nature of action bears striking relation to the idea of enacting embodiment. She notes:

> Action and speech go on between [wo]men .... Most action and speech is concerned with this in-between, which varies with each group of people, so that most words and deeds are about some worldly objective reality in addition to being a disclosure of the speaking and acting agent. (p. 182)

While many readers might problematize Arendt's positing of a "worldly objective reality" here, her focus in this passage is on the liminal space between humans in which we enact our identities and are conditioned by environmental aspects of the space—and I would add race, too. Moreover, this worldly objective reality, understood from a phenomenological orientation, is merely the "world-taken-for-granted"—that is, the world as it appears as "just there" and which we rely on in daily life in an unquestioned way—made to seem as if it is objective. Given that, as is well known, a dozen witnesses to any given accident or event will often have a dozen different recollections, our performative enactment of embodiment in this in-between space is likely to be diversely viewed and interpreted by others.

The second critical text that resonates in this regard and interrelates significantly with Titchkosky, is Butler's (1993) "Imitation and Gender Insubordination." In exploring the idea of fixed identity categories, Butler argues that these can open possibilities for both oppression and resistance, stating, "Identity categories tend to be instruments of regulatory regimes, whether as the normalizing categories of oppressive structures or as the rallying points for a liberatory contestation of that very oppression" (Butler, 1993, cited in Titchkosky, 2000, p. 208). Butler's insight allows people with disabilities to understand the possibilities of "re-colonizing" the identity categories and definitions that demarcate their lives and experiences. They contend that "identity categories are socially constructed and tend to be instruments of regulatory regimes" (Titchkosky, 2000, p. 308). In the context of this research, one of the most persuasive emancipatory potentials of Butler's argument lies in how they enable us to highlight these flawed categories to push for more inclusive freedoms. In Butler's words, "There remains a political imperative to use these necessary errors or category mistakes ... to rally and represent an oppressed political constituency" (p. 309). At the same time, however, Titchkosky's observation reminds us that while we may be interested in engaging in "liberatory contestation," we cannot ignore the fact that these identity categories have "real consequences for real people."

In the introduction to *Rethinking Normalcy*, Titchkosky and Michalko (2009) make the point that, in most cultures, disability has not been defined according to the self-definition of people with disabilities. For example, in Western cultures, institutional professions exercise this power in conceptualizing disability as a tragic problem:

> Despite the impossible belief that disability is not a broad social issue, there are still people and institutions that begin from the premise that disability is simply a rare and anomalous personal tragedy. It is precisely this "personal tragedy" conception of disability that acts as the impetus and provides the foundation for the study of disability. Professions such as medicine, rehabilitation, counselling, and special education have their own ways of defining disability .... What these professions share in common, however, is that disability is a personal tragedy wrought with problems, problems for which solutions must be sought. That disability is a personal problem of tragic proportions requiring the assistance of the helping professions makes this story the major one that disabled people in Western cultures are forced to inhabit today. (p. 2)

As Titchkosky and Michalko (2009) point out, the existence of these institutions that are able to define disability as a problem they seek to "cure" raises a seeming paradox, for while "this has led to a gigantic helping industry, it has not resulted in changing the marginalization and discrimination faced by disabled people on a daily basis" (p. 4). Identifying a similar problem, Hurst (1999) suggests, "Disabled people's own organizations happened as a direct action against the oppression of the medical rehabilitation professionals and psychiatrists, and their assumption that they 'owned' disability, and by inference, disabled people" (p. 25). From my personal experience and years of work in this field, I have found that the feeling among people with disabilities that they must resist being "owned" by institutions—whether by the medical establishment or government agencies such as the Ontario Disability Support Program—is both widely-held and deep. It is almost as if people with disabilities feel they are resisting a form of "slavery" whereby their bodies, and how their bodies are represented in cultural space, are being controlled or defined by others.

While this insight may seem obvious, I would argue that it is extraordinarily significant for understanding disability today. Consider its implications in reference to the news articles on PTSD. It is not surprising that the term "tragedy" or "tragedies" is used in articles and applied to people with PTSD, who are regarded as having a mental illness. It is very interesting to note that this usage is common among people in the "helping industry," medical professionals, and those making money off PTSD research and new therapies.

I should emphasize that in raising this point, I am not saying that scientific or medical research should not be supported and funded. What I do believe is important is the point highlighted by Titchkosky and Michalko (2009) above, that the existence of a "gigantic helping industry" with control over the definition of disability, invariably as a "tragic problem," has not resulted in any change in the marginalization of people with disabilities. In a sense, the industry needs people with disabilities to be "problem people" to justify, at least in part, their existence. The power to define something, to define people, is a very real power and not a thing that any institution will yield without a struggle (Butler, 1993; Foucault, 1995; Smith, 2005; Thomas, 1971; Titchkosky, 2024).

In considering my own experience with the PTSD diagnosis, the only "cure" I was informed about was medication for the treatment of symptoms. However, making medication the only cure meant that the cure was provisional and dependent upon institutional dispensing of medication and suggested that I would potentially never achieve "normalcy." In effect, I would always be a "problem person." This issue with fixed identity categories is a major reason people with disabilities are suspicious of identity politics and resistant to even claiming the social identifier of disability. As Garland-Thomson (2002) observes:

> The refusal to claim disability identity is in part due to a lack of ways to understand or talk about disability that are not oppressive …. Nonetheless, by disavowing disability identity, many of us learned to save ourselves from devaluation by a complicity that perpetuates oppressive notions. (p. 22)

Garland-Thomson's (2002) statement illustrates the complex double-bind confronting people with disability—the pervasiveness of social labeling and reduction of people with disabilities leaves few avenues to self-identification that are not oppressive; yet, avoiding self-identification can make one complicit in that same hegemonic and discriminatory order—and can remove access to resources that can help one achieve their goals. This position is not unlike that assumed by Butler (1993) when they noted their unease and anxiety with "being" a lesbian; that is, operating under the fixed identity category of lesbian or homosexual. In part, this stems from their unease at entering into a contest that may result in their being "recolonized" within this category. Butler also makes the point that this definitional struggle is related but exists apart from the reality of who they are as a subject.

Performance

Butler (1993) suggests that the representational field is a site of performance in which they perform being a lesbian as an identity category, but they explicitly caution that this does not exhaust or limit the reality of who they are as an "I." In Butler's words:

> When and where does this playing a lesbian constitute something like what I am? To say that I "play" at being one is not to say that I am not one "really" …. This is not a performance from which I can take radical distance, for this is deep-seated play …. What "performs" does not exhaust the "I"; it does not lay out in visible terms the comprehensive content of that "I." (p. 311)

Butler is addressing the distinction between "the Real and the Representational" (Garland-Thomson, 1997)—that is, between the raw experiences (sometimes confused) of people living with disability (such as myself) and the cultural representations of disability that can serve, at one and the same time, as discursive sites of oppression and resistance—as a performative space; that is, the making and defining of an identity category and the willingness to perform within this category as a political act while nonetheless emphasizing that this definition does not exhaust who one is as a subject. Fixed identity categories with respect to disability, as with gender or race, have always possessed a performative aspect:

> Race, gender, and sexual orientation may seem self-evidently fixed at birth, yet there is a strong "performative" element to the lived experience of identity. As the French philosopher Simone de Beauvoir famously wrote: "One is not born a woman, but, rather, becomes one." (Potolsky, 2006, p. 128)

Restated, while I may have a learning disability or PTSD, these are not what I am as a person, as a human being. While one may "perform" disability as a political act of resistance, contesting the power of institutional forces to recolonize the sign of "disability" by controlling its definition, one engages in this performance—even when it is "deep-seated play" with "real consequences for real people"—with recognition that it does not limit who one is.

Disability must be understood in terms of lives lived within the gap between the real and the representational. As we have tried to do for colonized people, so too should we understand the life experiences of disabled people through the eyes of the disabled; or, as second wave feminists put it, the "personal is political" (Hanisch, 2006, p. 1). Within disability studies, the connection of the personal and political is found in the disability activist phrase, "nothing about us without us," since disability status, including diagnosis and treatment, is not just personal but also political.

"The Performative is Political" is a self-conscious reference to the famous feminist activist slogan that is intended to highlight the political seriousness of the concept of "performing" in our discussion (Butler & Athanasiou, 2013; Hanisch, 2006). In everyday usage the term "performing" has connotations of theatricality and playing a role that is distinct from one's actual true self. In the context of this book, however, the concept of "performing" is theoretically grounded in cultural theories of political resistance to hegemonic authority with reference to Blackness, disability, and gender.

Framing the issue of PTSD within a critical disability studies perspective, and understanding the gap between the real and the representational, gives some illumination to my question of how to respond to this label of disability and its implications for my life. One possibility is opened by the contention that an individual can engage in an "identity" as a social performance in order to "pass" while at the same time attempting to isolate this from one's own sense of personal identity.

Feminist theory offers insights into how such a strategy may occur. As an example, feminist note that research conducted in the 1920s showed how women would engage in a "performance of womanliness" as a social defense mechanism (Potolsky, 2006). They argue that the attributes of femininity "could be assumed and worn as a mask" as a strategy for playing against, and resisting, the forces of social convention (Potolsky, 2006, p. 130). However, engaging in such contestations of power in terms of "fixed identity categories" is a clear and present danger and is arguably a reason many people with disabilities avoid engaging with the category of disability as much as possible.

With regard to disability, it is fascinating to note echoes of these perspectives in the words of Nancy Mairs's (1996) writing about how language—at the basic metaphorical level—alienates her from her body and defines her disability as shameful:

> The fact that the soundness of the body so often serves as a metaphor for moral health, its deterioration thus implying moral degeneracy, puts me and my kind in a quandary. How can I possibly be "good"? (p. 57)

As Titchkosky (2000) notes, it is important to recognize the "resources, institutional support, and authority" used by the "official text producers" in Western society to ideologically define the bodies of disabled people (p. 198). Moreover, the power of normalcy to "construct" disabled persons as non-normative can lead to stigmatization—which is a challenging and complex issue to address within Western society.

As Titchkosky (2000) writes, everyday practices, such as the use of language, "[encode] normalcy as the expected but taken for granted ground the 'we-the-normals' experience, an experience that does not usually obtrude upon one's consciousness. Instead, normalcy is the unmarked viewpoint from which deviance is observed" (p. 207). As both Titchkosky and Mairs (1996) point to, the pervasive power of the dominant culture—at the level of language itself—makes it extraordinarily challenging to develop strategies of resistance.

However, returning to women's performance of womanliness, a more complex analysis may suggest that women are subverting this same structure by using their agency in the way they select and deploy the attributes of "womanliness." This perspective is emphasized by the French feminist philosopher Luce Irigaray, who lays out a framework of gender performance as a strategy of resistance. Irigaray (1985) contends that women should play with the social conventions of femininity "without allowing themselves to be reduced to it" (p. 76). In this way, such a performance would undermine the claims of hegemonic social authority that being a "woman" was a matter of biological destiny and not, as Irigaray and other feminists contended, a social role.

These findings support the idea that this kind of passing is not only a feminist phenomenon but something that happens in many marginalized communities. The term "passing" is a fascinating concept that has had a long and contentious history for Black people. In a racial context, "passing" refers to people of one racially categorized group attempting to pass or be accepted as a member of another racial group. This form of passing is highly determined by social power relations in a society. Typically, it involves a person or group attempting to be accepted as a member of another particular group. In this book, passing is also a concept that is shaped, at its core, by an often-internalized awareness of social power relations. I would argue, therefore, that from a theoretical perspective, passing is a performance that is not necessarily dependent upon people believing one is not what one appears to be.

As Michalko (1998) observes, "The person who passes is aware of social situations and how they are interactionally produced and is thus always aware of what interaction is necessary to fit naturally into them" (p. 104). In other words, in order to pass, one must create an identity that is not quite one's "true" self or who they think or know their self to be—if such a thing can be said to exist—but is nonetheless a highly mediated relation between oneself and one's awareness of social expectations. In studies on passing among the disabled, researchers have found the same phenomenon (Evans, 2017; Heath-Stout, 2023; Prince, 2017; Samuels, 2003).

The phenomenon of passing also extends to Black people who are disabled. Research related to the phenomenon of passing among Black people has found that the marginalization they may experience in different social institutions, such as education and work, will motivate significant changes in the way they compensate for their positions so they appear "whiter" (Bahraini, 2021; DiAngelo, 2018; Fanon, 1967; Fordham, 1993). Indeed, inferiority is reinforced when the desire to imitate whiteness and white consciousness is felt by the oppressed group. For example, many Black people whiten their skin with skin bleaching products in an effort to have a lighter complexion so they can pass and throw off the burden of that corporeal malediction. Thus, the desire of many Black people to become whiter to pass reflects a deep-seated psychological and cultured alienation that is integral to Western civilization.

It is important to note that skin color means much more than pigmentation for Euro-Americans and Black people. For Euro-Americans, color signifies a vast range of cultural and psychological responses that are critical elements of the domination processes; for the colonized people, it signifies the desire to be like the colonizer. Unfortunately, many Black people do not realize that color is the most visible manifestation of their racial identity and altering it means erasing their natural identity. However, this is not restricted to Black people but extends to other colonized peoples as well.

A similar process of signifying the expected "ability" of the bodies and minds of citizens is found in dominant social and political discourses and images in media, in institutions, and in the material culture of the West, which constructs and presents Black or disabled bodies and minds as inferior and thus open to being oppressed by the rest of society, who then become a collective oppressor. It is notably difficult to resist and revolt against oppression when part of oneself believes the propaganda of the Euro-American oppression about one's inherent inferiority.

References

Agaibi, C. E., & Wilson, J. P. (2005). Trauma, PTSD, and resilience: A review of the literature. *Trauma, Violence, and Abuse*, 6(3), 195–216.

Alcoff, L. M. (1999). Toward a phenomenology of racial embodiment. *Radical Philosophy*, (95), 15–26.

American Psychiatric Association. (2000). *Diagnostic and statistical manual of mental disorders* (4th ed., text rev.).
Anand, S. (2020). Rethinking monsters: Teaching disability studies through history and the humanities. *Disability Studies in India: Interdisciplinary Perspectives*, 93–108.
Arendt, H. (1958). *The human condition*. University of Chicago Press.
Bahraini, A. (2021). The more ethnic the face, the more important the race: A closer look at colorism and employment opportunities among Middle Eastern women. *Humanity & Society, 45*(4), 617–637.
Bauman, Z. (2013). *Wasted lives: Modernity and its outcasts*. John Wiley & Sons.
Berger, R. J., & Wilbers, L. E. (2021). *Introducing disability studies* (2nd ed.). Lynne Rienner Publishers.
Bloche, M. G. (2011). *The hippocratic myth*. Macmillan.
Butler, J., & Athanasiou, A. (2013). Dispossession: *The performative in the political*. John Wiley & Sons.
Butler, J. (1993). Imitation and gender insubordination. In H. Abelove, M. Barale, & D. Halperin (Eds.), *The lesbian and gay studies reader* (pp. 307–320). Routledge.
Carter, R. T., Kirkinis, K., & Johnson, V. E. (2020). Relationships between trauma symptoms and race-based traumatic stress. *Traumatology, 26*(1), 11.
Chemtob, C., Roitblat, H. L., Hamada, R. S., Carlson, J. G., & Twentyman, C. T. (1988). A cognitive action theory of post-traumatic stress disorder. *Journal of Anxiety Disorders, 2*(3), 253–275.
Clegg, S. R., Courpasson, D., & Phillips, N. (2006). *Power and organizations*. Pine Forge Press.
Cohen, J., Friedman, M., Keane, T., & Foa, E. (2009). *Effective treatments for PTSD: Practice guidelines from the international society for traumatic stress studies*. Guildford Publications.
Davis, L. J. (1995). *Enforcing normalcy: Disability, deafness, and the body*. Verso Books.
Davis, L. (2013). *The end of normal: Identity in a biocultural era*. University of Michigan Press.
DiAngelo, R. (2018). *White fragility: Why it's so hard for white people to talk about racism*. Beacon Press.
Engel, S., & Logan, N. (2013, November 29). Soldier suicides prompt concerns about military mental health support. *Global News*. https://globalnews.ca/news/999826/soldier-suicides-prompt-concerns-about-military-mental-health-support/.
Evans, H. D. (2017). Un/covering: Making disability identity legible. *Disability Studies Quarterly, 37*(1).
Everly, J. G. S., & Lating, J. M. (2013). *A clinical guide to the treatment of the human stress response*. Springer.
Fanon, F. (1967). *Black skin, white masks*. Trans. Charles Lam Markmann. Grove Press.
Fordham, S. (1993). Those loud black girls: (Black) women, silence, and gender "passing" in the academy. *Anthropology & Education Quarterly, 24*(1), 3–32.
Foucault, M. (1995). *Discipline and punish: The birth of the prison*. Trans. Alan Sheridan. Random House.

Garland-Thomson, R. (1997). *Extraordinary bodies: Figuring physical disability in American culture and literature.* Columbia University Press.
Garland-Thomson, R. (2002). Integrating disability, transforming feminist theory. *NWSA Journal, 14*(3), 1–32.
Garland-Thomson, R. (2020). Integrating disability, transforming feminist theory. In *Feminist theory reader* (pp. 181–191). Routledge.
Goodley, D. (2013). Dis/entangling critical disability studies. *Disability & Society, 28*(5), 631–644.
Goodley, D. (2014). *Dis/ability studies: Theorising disablism and ableism.* Routledge.
Hanisch, C. (2006). *The personal is political: The women's liberation movement classic with a new explanatory introduction.* http://webhome.cs.uvic.ca/~mserra/AttachedFiles/PersonalPolitical.pdf.
Heath-Stout, L. E. (2023). The invisibly disabled archaeologist. *International Journal of Historical Archaeology, 27*(1), 17–32.
Hurst, R. (1999). Disabled people's organisations and development: Strategies for change. In E. Stone (Ed.), *Disability and development: Learning from action and research on disability in the majority world* (pp. 25–35). Disability Press.
Irigaray, L. (1985). *This sex which is not one.* Trans. C. Porter & C. Burke. Cornell University Press.
Johanssen, J., & Garrisi, D. (Eds.). (2020). *Disability, media, and representations: Other bodies.* Routledge.
Levinas, E. (1969). *Totality and infinity. An essay on exteriority.* Trans. Alphonso Lingis. Duquesne University Press.
Low, J. (1996). Negotiating identities, negotiating environments: An interpretation of the experiences of students with disabilities. *Disability & Society, 11*(2), 235–248.
Mairs, N. (1996). *Waist-high in the world: A life among the non-disabled.* Beacon Press.
McGuire, A. (2010). Disability, non-disability and the politics of mourning: Rethinking the "we." *Disability Studies Quarterly, 30*(3/4).
Michalko, R. (1998). *The mystery of the eye and the shadow of blindness.* University of Toronto Press.
Michalko, R. (2002). *The difference that disability makes.* Temple University Press.
Michalko, R. (2009). The excessive appearance of disability. *International Journal of Qualitative Studies in Education, 22*(1), 65–74.
Potolsky, M. (2006). *Mimesis.* Routledge.
Prince, M. J. (2017). Persons with invisible disabilities and workplace accommodation: Findings from a scoping literature review. *Journal of Vocational Rehabilitation, 46*(1), 75–86.
Roberson, K., & Carter, R. T. (2022). The relationship between race-based traumatic stress and the Trauma Symptom Checklist: Does racial trauma differ in symptom presentation? *Traumatology, 28*(1), 120.
Samuels, E. J. (2003). My body, my closet: Invisible disability and the limits of coming-out discourse. *GLQ: A Journal of Lesbian and Gay Studies, 9*(1), 233–255.
Schroeder-Lein, G. R. (2008). *The encyclopedia of civil war medicine.* New York, NY: M.E.

Sharpe. War Office of Great Britain. (1922). *Report of the War Office Committee of Enquiry into "Shell-shock."* London, U.K.: Imperial War Museum.

Schroeder-Lein, G. R. (2015). *The encyclopedia of civil war medicine.* Routledge.

Smith, D. E. (2005). *Institutional ethnography: A sociology for people.* AltaMira Press.

Taylor, S. (2011). Beasts of burden: Disability studies and animal rights. *Qui Parle: Critical Humanities and Social Sciences, 19*(2), 191–222.

Thomas, W. I. (1971). On the definition of the situation. In M. Truzzi (Ed.), *Sociology: The classic statements* (pp. 274–277). Random House. (Original work published 1923)

Titchkosky, T. (2000). Disability studies: The old and the new. *Canadian Journal of Sociology, 25*(2), 197–224.

Titchkosky, T. (2005). Disability in the news: A reconsideration of reading. *Disability & Society, 20*(6), 655–668. https://journals-scholarsportal-info.myaccess.library.utoronto.ca/pdf/09687599/v20i0006/655_ditnaror.xml.

Titchkosky, T. (2007). *Reading and writing disability differently: The textured life of embodiment.* University of Toronto Press.

Titchkosky, T. (2024). Interpretive methods in disability studies: Dyslexia inflected inquiry. *Qualitative Inquiry, 0*(0). https://doi.org/10.1177/10778004241254394.

Titchkosky, T., & Michalko, R. (2009). *Rethinking normalcy: A disability studies reader.* Canadian Scholars' Press.

Williams, M. T., Khanna Roy, A., MacIntyre, M. P., & Faber, S. (2022). The traumatizing impact of racism in Canadians of colour. *Current Trauma Reports, 8*(2), 17–34.

Williams, M. T., Printz, D., & DeLapp, R. C. (2018). Assessing racial trauma with the trauma symptoms of discrimination scale. *Psychology of Violence, 8*(6), 735.

Withuis, J. (2008). Introduction. In J. Withuis & A. Mooij (Eds.), *The politics of war trauma* (pp. 1–12). Amsterdam University Press.

World Health Organization and The World Bank. (2011). World report on disability. Retrieved from: http://www.who.int/disabilities/world_report/2011/en/index.html.

World Health Organization. (2023). Disability. Retrieved from https://www.who.int/health-topics/disability#tab=tab_3.

Chapter 3

Intersectionality

My experience can only be understood at a crossroads, the intersection between the cultural understanding of disability as "brokenness," the colonized Black body, and the performance of masculinity. The experience of disability is often an intersectional one, an experience that necessitates theoretical flexibility and multiple interpretive frames to more effectively understand the cultural production of Blackness and disability in our societies.

The concept of intersectionality was introduced by Kimberlé Crenshaw (1989) in an examination of the experiences of Black women's struggle against racism and systems of social oppression. Crenshaw argued that a single-axis analysis was insufficient and true insight into common experiences would be gained through a multidimensional review of both the racial aspects of discrimination in the Black experience and the female subjugation that was the progenitor of the feminist movement (p. 139).

The examination of the common experiences of the students will provide insight into their encounters with the university, their conflicts with regard to both accommodation and the discrimination that, according to both law and policy, they should not be encountering but that nonetheless exacerbates these individuals' marginalization. At the intersection of Blackness and disability, many experiences of marginalization are revealed that cannot be due to one's status as either a racial minority or a person with a disability. As I noted in the introduction, exploring the complexity of Blackness and disability can reveal the unique phenomenon of intersectional marginalization and its implications.

The concept of intersectionality as explored by disability scholar Titchkosky (2007) allows us to understand the complexity of marginalization and how the process of identifying disability and Blackness is deployed institutionally. She explains that within this process, marginalization and oppression can often be difficult to interpret. Sociologist Bauman (2004) states that "wars of recognition" that seek to define identities are subject to marginalization and oppression (p. 35), but he also points out that these identities are not always solid. Their fluidity manifests especially on ethical grounds when we interpret other groups as deficient, less free, or less moral. Disability studies, for example, is certainly embedded in this construction and deployment of normalcy that animates the assumption about what one should have the "ability" to do or to what degree one is free from being overdetermined by physical or mental conditions.

Titchkosky (2007) further observes—with reference to the discursive analysis of disability and to Blackness through Butler's (2004) concept of "recognition"—that it is obvious that our culture does not, in the main, recognize disability as having a "viable" status: "Butler theorizes the social act of recognition, in which some people are recognized as less than human and produced as non-viable" (Titchkosky, 2007, p. 6). Titchkosky is suggesting that disability discourse serves something other than the interests of people with disabilities: "Disability is made viable as a metaphor to express only that which is unwanted and that which is devastatingly inept" (p. 5; see also Iannacci & Graham, 2010). This raises the question: Why?

To address this question, we can make use of the theoretical concept of intersectionality (Titchkosky, 2007, p. 3) and how we make meaning at the intersecting differences of our identities. For instance, when

Titchkosky (2007) argues that "viable status is not granted to disability" (p. 6), she is highlighting how difference remains fundamentally unacknowledged in Western culture. At its signifying core, difference remains fundamentally alien to Western culture. Disability and Blackness are often represented not just as a diminishment or a departure from a normative standard but as something radically alien within our culture and thus, often, subject to taboo. In addressing Titchkosky's statement above, we can make use of the theoretical model of intersectionality to explain how we make meaning at the intersecting differences of our identities.

Given this complex context of recognition, misrecognition, and a failure to imagine, I proffer that it is only through an inclusive theoretical and cultural apparatus that we can come to understand the full complexity of disability, marginality, and the potential for resistance. As hooks (1990) notes in her commentary on using one's marginalization as a form of resistance:

> When Bob Marley sings, "We refuse to be what you want us to be, we are what we are, and that's the way it's going to be," that space of refusal, where one can say no to the colonizer, no to the downpressor, is located in the margins. (p. 341)

From this perspective, hooks' (1990) theoretical engagement with the meaning of marginality can be used to make sense of the strategies of students with disabilities who resist the foreclosure of their future education possibilities based on the limited significations that are applied to their social identities. These identities are eclipsed in social space, and in theoretical constructs, highlighting the limitations of theoretical models in attending to their Blackness and disability.

To explore marginalization, I will discuss scholarship connecting disability and race in the contemporary context to illustrate how "normal" and "disabled" bodies must be understood in terms of social power (Davis, 2020; Demetriou & Symeonidou, 2021; Titchkosky & Michalko, 2009). Medical and social models of disability will be defined—this research operates from the theoretical perspective of the latter—to better understand how this process of marginalization has and continues to define Blackness and disability in an inequitable way.

As Garland-Thomson (2002) states, "Disability theory's most incisive critique is revealing the intersections between the politics of appearance and the medicalization of subjugated bodies" (p. 10). This means that the bodies of those that are "different" are treated as something problematic. Therefore, they are thought to be in need of medical care and maintenance. In this sense, the bodies of the disabled are marked as being inferior.

Another way in which disabled bodies have been constructed as inferior is through the political economy. In particular, the colonialist mode of production has resulted in a distinctive response to disability. Indeed, I assert that this is an especially critical point in exploring this experience of disability, as the following events occurred at an interpretative crossroads that had the effect of obscuring, for many years, my understanding of the role of disability in my experience.

While scholars have long noted the parallels between Blackness and disability-based prejudice, one aspect of this common experience is only recently attracting critical attention: the complex cultural anxiety with regard to Black masculinity and disability (Erevelles, 2019; Pickens, 2021). In Jamaica and Canada, the history of institutional discursive practices in relation to the sexuality of Black men as well as people with disabilities can be seen as closely intertwined.

One way they are intertwined is under the cultural assumptions that ground the objective of disciplining bodies deemed deviant within common culture. As one scholar (Jarman, 2012) writes, for both groups their "nonconforming sexuality functioned as a foundational indicator of otherness and was deployed … to secure the public's approval of medical regulation and confinement" to control what both institutional and popular discourses represented as the "sexual promiscuity" and "excessive appetites" of Black men and people with disabilities (p. 96).

Both Black masculinity and disabled persons have been and remain objects of cultural fear and sites of deviance. It is important, from the outset, to define the theoretical, political, and personal origins for the exploration of the discourses of Blackness and disability in our culture. In making an argument about intertwined cultural anxieties with relation to Black masculinity and disability, I do not mean to subordinate one to the other in any respect. Thus, while I hold that Blackness and disability have operated in Western culture as distinct discourses, I agree with Jarman (2012) that these discourses also function "fluidly" and are "often employed to undergird one another" (p. 92).

For example, in the context of my Jamaican experience of disability, as a child, I did not understand how my body had already been inscribed by complex historical forces born of the colonial legacy. In my own volunteer work with unhoused people in Toronto, I know very well how "material" issues of race, Blackness, masculinity, disability, and class play critical roles in the experience and definition of being unhoused.

Commentators have noted that the use of the human body as an inscriptive surface upon which to "write" a vast range of messages is a phenomenon that stretches back in time to the very origins of human society itself (Grosz, 2009). Of course, it is possible to reference numerous examples of such inscriptions encountered in the public sphere on a daily basis. Humans seem to have a predisposition toward marking ourselves and inscribing—sometimes through contested processes of "reading"—different meanings upon the bodies of others.

For example, young people may inscribe themselves with hip-hop clothing and styling that reflect "masculine culture" to project a message of strength—a message that can be read, from other perspectives, as an inscription of self-marginalization or of bravado masking a lack of self-confidence. What is occurring here, I will argue, is what Foucault (1988) might call a "technique of self-production" (as cited in Grosz, 2009, p. 143).

However, the key question relates to the "very status of the body as product—the question is whose product?" (Grosz, 2009, p 143). This latter form is, I would argue, particularly significant. As Grosz (2009) notes, less openly violent but no less coercive are the inscriptions of cultural and personal values, norms, and commitments according to the morphology and categorization of the body into socially significant groups—male and female, Black and white, and so on. Nonetheless, people in either Jamaica or Canada, or any cultural frame, constitute their identities and sense of the world at the intersection of differences.

In terms of my own experience, while I initially interpreted my disability in terms of masculinity, I came to understand it in terms of

Blackness and disability and eventually as a cultural mélange of all three marginalizing social positionings. In this context, I argue that it is not only through an inclusive theoretical and cultural apparatus that we can come to understand the full complexity of the disability, marginality, and potential for resistance in our society.

It is also important to engage in inductive reasoning and introspection regarding the experiences of others. All people have a story, and it is important to understand their story and what it means within these frameworks. This work demonstrates that when we are able to situate ourselves in the colonialist discourses that permeate our culture, we are better able to address the complexities and issues of our culture and understand how to create a more equitable human society in the years to come.

Academic approaches to the intersection of Blackness and disability have been varied. Critical theorists' complex works depict colonialism as a set of processes that involve not only physical struggle but also psychological and pedagogical struggles as well as cultural marginalization (Dei, 2017; Pickens, 2017). Some theorists have treated certain categories of difference as simply nuances of other categories. For example, one criticized stance is that of treating the oppression of Black women as simply a nuanced version of the marginalization of women. Erevelles and Minear (2010) argue that disability faces a similar challenge: it is often relegated to the status of nuance rather than an identity category in itself. Yet, it will be shown that being Black and disabled often results in more than the sum of the challenges inherent in each identity.

The idea of racial inferiority is grounded in the same principle of departure from a "normal" state as disability (Erevelles & Minear, 2010, p. 133). In the educational system, a significantly larger proportion of students who are labeled as disabled or who have difficulty learning are Black than white. Erevelles and Minear (2010) view this as a particular form of marginalization. Blackness can thus exacerbate problems associated with exclusion and marginality in the case of Black individuals with learning difficulties. However, conditions in marginalized communities often do not accommodate variant ability and thus contribute to learning and behavioral problems stemming from disabilities

(Erevelles & Minear, 2010, pp. 137–139). Being Black and disabled are two categorical differences that exist on their own but also inform each other in particular ways when they are present in the same individual.

Being Black and disabled on campus often breeds conflicts for students in those situations. Many of them are conflicted about disclosure or passing. If they reveal their identity, they stand to get accommodations, which will make their life easier. On the other hand, if they expose their hidden disabilities, like attention deficit disorder, anxiety, or depression, their peers may look at them differently. Disclosure is perceived as a double-edged sword because it leads to discrimination and social distancing. Trammell (2009) calls this "wearing the red shirt." Telling others that one has a mental illness is highly risky. Students have to do a cost-benefit analysis of which decision has fewer dangers. When one is Black, their marginal racial identity and the stereotypes associated with being Black are amalgamated with disabilities to make their experiences in campus extremely difficult.

Numerous stereotypes are associated with being Black and being disabled in university. Mentally ill people are often perceived as incompetent and dangerous. When an institution relied on the medical model of disability, the social stigma continues to be worse since the model of mental illness worsens social stigma. Likewise, the same is true for being Black. As mentioned before, many Black students face negative reactions from their non-Black peers who stereotype them as dangerous (Jamil, 2022). When these race-based stereotypes are combined with stereotypes around mental illness, their experiences become grim (Mayor, 2023). In other words, by stigmatizing a certain human trait, associating a negative stereotype with it, and responding to students based on those responses means that educational experiences are vastly compromised for Black students with disabilities.

The Politics of Identity

The students who participated in the study that informs this book all self-identified as Black students with a disability. The students had in common their Blackness and that they are navigating the complexities of university life as disabled individuals. In the interviews, I was particularly interested in the convergence of these two "defining" characteristics. Their sometimes varied but sometimes common experiences will illustrate the practical application of the Ontario Human Rights Code with regards to persons with disabilities. Because I am interested in this institutional understanding of disability, when I use the defining identification of "disabled," it is in the context of the body of legislation, rules, and administrative interpretations thereof not as a descriptor of the individual.

Disability continuously exists as part of an interconnected identity that encompasses race, sex, sexuality, class, and gender presentation, with categories informing each other (Pickens, 2017). Thus, analyzing them demands defining how audiences and people with disabilities accept or manipulate the narrative. Blackness and disability do not always disappear from the narrative view as problems solved in narratives focusing on Black disabled people; they or others fail to consider them as problems. Pickens (2017) emphasizes that discussions focusing on Blackness and disability fail to erase disability and Blackness; however, they still make meaning irrespective of their focus.

Disability identity is political owing to the dominant narratives and how people with disabilities themselves interpret their situations. Some students with disabilities choose to love what others hate (Folb, 2013). Adults with dyslexia, for example, may choose to perceive the condition as a different way of thinking rather some sort of flaw. In the university and educational environment, it is perceived as a negative thing to be regulated (Sagar et al., 2024; Michalko & Titchkosky, 2024). Therefore, some dyslexics prefer not to identify with other dyslexics. People with the condition thus wind up treating their peers in the same discriminatory way that society has treated them. They have gone with the dominant position. Nonetheless, certain individuals break away from that narrative.

The institutions themselves may undermine people's ability to claim the disability label. In some higher educational institutions, it is not enough for one to use poor performance as a justification of their need for accommodations. Accessibility offices depend on the medical disability model, which pathologizes disability (Anderson, 2023). There is a needs hierarchy, which is driven by ableist ideas. Therefore, higher educational institutions frame disability in terms of functional limitation. On the other hand, some persons with disabilities perceive it as a social construction so they may not identify with that label.

Sometimes the need for self-sufficiency and independence causes Black students with disabilities to claim they are not disabled. Toutain (2019) found that many of these students wanted to be independent. Therefore, using accommodations would make them seem like they are not. Some students on campus only use accommodations as backup and instead prefer to carry on without any support from the administration. Some even justified it by saying they were not going to receive the same accommodations in the real world beyond college, so there was no point in getting accustomed to it. This sentiment stems from the highly individualist nature of the West. Society prioritizes individual abilities, so students with disabilities who depended on the accommodations of others felt like their success was diluted by the contributions of others (Jackson, 2022). A person's work tends to be valued more the less accommodations they have. Therefore, this makes people hide who they are.

Certain individuals do not want to identify with their disability status because of tokenism. Cameron and Jefferies (2021) explain that it is complicated for students with disabilities because many of them do not have the support they require to succeed in school, but at the same time, these individuals are selected for copious amounts of committee work, as the token marginalized member, which they are encouraged to do to support the community of persons of color with disabilities. However, a significant number of people are not happy with those outcomes.

As Saga clearly stated when I asked him about his disability, "I ain't disabled." I further questioned Saga, "How do you access accommodations with the Accessibility Services Office if you are not 'disabled'?" His reply succinctly encapsulated the general experience: that he has accepted this societal label as a means to access the needed, and legally mandated, accommodations that allow him to adapt the university environment and educational structure to his unique form of comprehension. He added, "My disability is 'invisible.' I have a learning disability, what we now call 'invisible' disability. What is a 'normal' person"? If we consider this response, Saga's comment about being "invisible" can take on a new meaning. It could be that the more "troubling" the disability, the greater the interest of society in keeping the person invisible. Consider, for example, the phenomena of segregation and institutionalization of arguably the most extreme examples in the history of Western society of the exclusion of those branded deviant from the general population (Malacrida, 2016; Ferri & Connor, 2006). While Saga's highly "visible" Blackness and the assumption it causes others to mark him with needles even with his invisible disability.

In the famous African American book, Ellison's *Invisible Man* (1952), the experience of African Americans is likened to being an "invisible" population in American discourse. As Ellison writes:

> I am an invisible man. No, I am not a spook like those who haunted Edgar Allan Poe; nor am I one of your Hollywood-movie ectoplasms. I am a man of substance, of flesh and bone, fiber, and liquids—and I might even be said to possess a mind. I am invisible, understand, simply because people refuse to see me. Like the bodiless heads you see sometimes in circus sideshows, it is as though I have been surrounded by mirrors of hard distorting glass. When they approach me, they see only my surroundings, themselves, or figments of their imagination—indeed, everything and anything except me. (p. 3)

Ellison's illustrative anecdote is particularly fascinating because it highlights how invisibility is equated with the power to marginalize Black bodies. However, we can see the significant implications of his depiction of the body problem that may be termed the "colonized body." In this chapter, Césaire's (1972) deconstruction of colonialism and Goffman's (1967) theory of human interactions allow us to understand how the "invisible body" represented in Ellison's story is a "colonized body." Does the "colonization of the body" in contemporary Western society make us all complicit in this process? According to Fanon's (1967) psychological analysis, the effects of colonial Europeans' control of thought industries made Black or disabled persons accept their colonized, subordinate position as natural. Ellison explains that he is an invisible man simply because others refuse to see him. Indeed, these are feelings that remain with Black disabled students, particularly those who require academic accommodations.

It may be speculated that Saga's success in his performance of disability was due, at least in part, to his being at the intersection of multiple social oppressions—Blackness, disability, class, and masculinity. From this experience, Saga expresses an intuitive understanding of oppression that can develop as a part of one's everyday lived experience at that intersection. Perhaps, as Butler (1993), Garland-Thomson (1997), and other critics suggest, the success of such performances can lie in the attributes one chooses to deploy.

It is noteworthy that people with disabilities—much like Black individuals in their performance of racialized identities—resist how hegemonic cultural forces in Western society have traditionally sought to foreclose their identities within a narrow frame. While our bodies have an obvious corporeal or physical existence, they exist in arguably more complex and multifarious ways in "cultural encoding" comprised of both "conventions of representation and the complexities of identity production without social narratives of bodily differences" (Garland-Thomson, 1997, p. 5). As one critic observes, while the cultural encoding can be complex, the output of this process is almost invariably reductionist: "Disability cancels out other qualities, reducing the complex person to a single attribute" (Garland-Thomson, 1997, p. 12).

Garland-Thomson (1997) asks that we consider how easily one can replace "disability" with "race" in the sentence. Thus, instead of: "Disability cancels out other qualities, reducing the complex person to a single attribute" we have: "Race cancels out other qualities, reducing the complex person to a single attribute." As we toggle between these distinct yet very closely related sentences, it allows us to understand the theoretical proximity of "disability" and "race" in this chapter. Performing disability may nonetheless be regarded as a valuable strategy as it offers us a means by which people with disabilities can improvise, assimilate, and re-deploy the needed markers of disability that hegemonic social authority uses to limit the identities of people with disabilities as a way of asserting their "own" identity in everyday life. Moreover, the performance of disability can be considered a strategy of economy that enables individuals—with a minimal array of gestures and improvisations—to optimize their life experiences and resist the foreclosure or reduction of identity by hegemonic social forces in our culture.

In attempting to problematize this construction and performance of lived identities and issues of social stigma, passing, and social hierarchies, I rely on the work of disability theorists such as Michalko (1998), who, in his discussion of the concept of "passing," placing particular emphasis on what Goffman (1967) refers to as "impression management." In other words, a blind person who is attempting to "pass" as sighted must become a skillful social actor capable of "calculative and attentive interaction." The critical issue here is one of "stigma."

As Michalko (1998) notes with regard to rehabilitation from disability, "Rehabilitation is fundamentally interested in the restoration of a condition or status in which, before restoration, one lives in degradation … or, as Goffman (1963) might say, a 'stigma'" (p. 69). In a sense, as with all performances of the self, this is a performance of a highly complex order in that one is playing dual overlapping roles; both oneself and a "passing" persona. Again, as with all performances of the self in social settings, this dual role is significant. As Butler (1993) notes vis-à-vis their own social performances of gender: "This is not a performance from which I can take radical distance, for this is deep-seated play, psychically entrenched play" (p. 311).

From the outset, it must be acknowledged that the concept of "performance" is contested in the sense that its precise definition is notably elusive. A strong argument has been made by a number of theorists and critics that performance can, by definition, encompass a wide range of human social behaviors in which actions are intended to influence others in the social relationship (Schechner, 2006). Thus, the concept of performance has come to be applied to an extraordinarily diverse range of human activities and behaviors. In this regard, Butler's (1993) concept of performativity is particularly useful in the analysis. They contend that performativity is

> Not a [single] "act," for it is always a reiteration of a norm or set of norms …. Moreover, this act is not primarily theatrical; indeed, its apparent theatricality is produced to the extent that its historicity remains dissimulated. (p. 12)

Butler's (1993) discussion of performativity is informed by their focus on issues of gender construction and, in particular, how heterosexuality is constructed by discursive power as a normative human condition. Butler's understanding of performativity may be usefully applied to the role of Black disabled students in their performance, especially since they argue that performativity enables the "recasting of the matter of bodies as the effect of a dynamic of power, such that the matter of bodies will be indissociable from the regulatory norms that govern their materialization and the signification of those material effects" (p. 2). Michalko (1998) has noted that these performances are all interactional, as the self is created in the space between people. As Titchkosky (2007) notes with reference to the appearances of disability, these are "enactments" of "social life .... The meaning of disability lies 'between' people and not merely in people" (pp. 17–18).

In assessing such an enactment, as one critic observes, we must focus on the intersections of the categories of disability, Blackness, gender, and class: "Wherever social stratification exists—and it is evident in all complex societies—gender, race [Blackness] and disability are ... carried in the broader class structure" (Meekosha, 2006, p. 171). In this case, I argue that Saga's decision to claim the disability he otherwise disavows achieved him the desired end because it contained enough multilayered symbolic volume that it overrode the everyday filters or "blinders" that most people have with regard to disability.

Titchkosky's statement above echoes Walcott's (1996) discussion of the performance of "Blackness" with reference to self and expressive cultural practices, such as rap and hip-hop. It can be seen to have clear associations with the theorizing of appearance and performance of disability. All of this raises the question: Why do people—whether they have disabilities or are Black—attempt to pass? Michalko (1998) addresses this by using the highly allusive metaphor of shadow: "Blindness becomes a mere shadow of its former status .... There is a qualitative and quantitative difference between the self and its shadow" (p. 67). Michalko is here commenting on the moral character of rehabilitation that informs the socially accepted view that the condition of sight is the normative state of being and blindness is its shadow, a condition of lower status. Such a conception influences what can and cannot be learned about disability and disability identity and ultimately has an influence on how any "social change" does or does not make an appearance.

These differences are significant and, I will argue, shape the objectives of people with disabilities and Black people who attempt to pass. In a sense, passing can be seen to be an act of resistance to exclusion. From this perspective, it is understandable why people with disabilities would seek to "pass" as people without disabilities. Given the pervasiveness of prevailing social discourse—together with the fact that we build our "self" interactively and so cannot easily ignore dominant social expectations—it is clear why many would prefer to take this route, if possible. Of course, this opens the door to discussion about what is an "essential" self, even in a social context. Certainly, I will argue that the performance of Blackness—in its complexity—has clear parallels with the performance of disability, as referenced in *The Mystery of the Eye and the Shadow of Blindness* (Michalko, 1998). There is resistance to being tagged with an actual label and the associated negative implications and stigmatization establishes a baseline of tension.

The assumption in the process is that students are passive receptacles—they are what Foucault (1995) refers to as "docile bodies." He notes that:

> docile bodies rely heavily on the way social institutions and various power centers use discipline and control one's individuality. The docility of a body is forged through the various disciplinary measures that are usually applied to limit the actions of a person within the regulated norms (p. 47).

This type of discipline is often defined through the slow and deliberate measures that are part of how powerful individuals access the human body, as well as how they integrate their norms to isolate and categorize a particular person. Foucault (1995) defines this type of discipline through the creation of docility within the individual:

> Thus, discipline produces subjected and practiced bodies; docile bodies. Discipline increases the forces of the body (in economic terms of utility) and diminishes these same forces (in political terms of obedience). In short, it dissociates power from the body. (p. 138)

Through the direct manipulation of the body, the agent power ascertains the nature of the mental function of the student by creating these obstacles to their individuality. The "dissociation" of self is part of this physic exertion of force that enables the ultimate political docility and the apathy that results. This is one important aspect of how power seeks to make the body submissive through institutional means and, therefore, brings about the physic apathy that makes a body docile to the maintenance of that power. Within the large social scale, the docile body is important for people who experience power. The instruments of discipline master the physical and eventually dominate the mental competence of those subject to it.

A critical analysis of Blackness and disability in the university reveals issues beyond labeling and stigmatization of students. The significant differences in the definition of Blackness and disability in university settings provides critical evidence of the fact that disability, like race, is not a physical given but a cultural construct. By the late twentieth century, it had become widely acknowledged in both scholarly and popular environments that "labeling" people with a particular "identity" is not only inaccurate but also often harmful to both the subject and the wider society (Galinsky et al., 2003). For example, Black students who are labeled as disabled not only face challenges stemming from their disability but also face institutional consequences of this double categorization (Grant & An, 2021). With respect to Blackness or disability—among the most powerful stigmas in Western culture—it has become accepted that labeling can have an adverse impact on how a person sees themselves and how others will see them.

Back et al. (2016) investigated the issue of labeling students with disabilities in a U.S. urban school district. Their study focused on expressing an understanding of the nature of disability and the implications it has for the identity of people in the system. The conflict under investigation in the study was the difference between disability-first and people-first language and how it is that research could contribute to understanding the specific linguistic implications on personality and the way that disabled people saw themselves. The conclusion was that it is important that schools move toward creating an improved language for dealing with individuals with disabilities as well as toward the development of a positive disability identity. Achieving this would be important, especially in communities where there is intersectional marginalization of citizens such as urban settings, where both Black and disabled people will more commonly live and where there will be several Black disabled people. In this sense, labeling has negative implications for people who are Black or disabled in the education system; however, it is an ongoing process (Back et al., 2016; Smith, 1982).

In understanding this process, it is important to recognize not only oppressive social constructions of the self across time but also of revolutionary theory and practice that resists these very constructions. As we have seen in following this thread across decades of intellectual thought and political/social struggle, this social construction of the self is often deployed to reinforce a social/political hierarchy through the association of qualities of inferiority/superiority and normative/deviance with categorization of physical bodies.

This critical analysis also demonstrates that Black identity matters to the formulation of disability studies because it brings some of these ideas about the "other" and normalizing powers to the discussion. It also matters because it provides a space wherein Black disabled students are able to articulate their racial identities without being subsumed under this general category of "being" disabled. This is both a cultural and political point because it recognizes that marginalized voices can be differentiated and also united under a common goal, and thus it creates a critical place for thinking about inclusion.

Therefore, as I have argued, it is not sufficient to rely wholly upon post-modern disavowals of stable identity because there needs to be some space for racial identity to be expressed so that people do not feel subjected to the same old "gazes" that DuBois (1903) (and hooks, 1992) revealed and interrogated. There is much to learn from these voices, which have deep roots in a historical struggle for awareness, recognition, and identity inclusion.

When conducting studies concerning the treatment of marginalized groups, one aspect of social identity that is essential is its outward manifestation and observability by outsiders or vested parties. In this case, these identity traits are often taken to occupy distinct though sometimes ambiguous categories: the visible, the invisible, and the non-visible. In general terms, the visible and invisible refer to physical qualities and quantities of the identity of the individual (Alcoff, 2006, p. 11), and in this research, to Blackness and disability. The non-visible is attributed to the mental state or self-affiliation of the identity of the individual, often sexual orientation, political persuasion, or personal philosophy traits that cannot be tested for through physical means.

The facts of visibility and invisibility factored prominently into the responses (seen or unseen) of the students. The students spoke of their Blackness being readily apparent for their peers and professors to judge and make assumptions on; however, many had disabilities that were "hidden or invisible" and only by virtue of using Accessibility Services and having academic accommodations were their disabilities known. Zaine, a second year master's student, stated, "My disability, given that it is invisible in nature, makes it difficult for people to identify what is 'wrong' with me." The learning disabilities and their revelation through accommodations resulted in much of the stigmatization spoken of earlier.

Fuligni (2007) illustrates that standard school practices, including instructors' labeling and social groups and segregation, trigger the tendencies of students to categorize, label, stereotype, and rank other learners on different qualities, such as academic abilities and potential. Group dynamics impact how students interpret explicit and implicit curricular messages regarding social groups (Pierre, 2012). According to Fuligni (2007), students labeled as inferior often behave as inferior, whereas those labeled as superior perform in a consistently superior manner. Social identities and attitudes can also influence students' schooling, and at the same time, their experiences in school can influence their social identities and attitudes. This exercise is convincing because the student had never thought about eye color as a significant aspect of the self or a foundation for discriminating against others. In addition, it takes only a few messages to influence students' self-conceptions, feelings toward their peers, and educational performance.

The explicit use of gender to label students and organize the settings is integral to the etiology of gender stereotyping. This type of labeling is also common among Black students with disabilities seeking accommodations for their studies, especially those with mental illnesses

(Mintz & Fraser, 2024). Changing historical racial constraints on Black status supports collective identity and offers the context for comprehending why Black students label and avoid some attitudes and behaviors as "white" (Fuligni, 2007). Changing ideas of how white people expected Black students to act and react or risk punishment reflects the changing racial constraints. In response, Black people developed ways of being that were expressed in opposition to these white expectations.

Disability labels, including mental illness, PTSD, and intellectual disability, have been connected to racially changed meanings. Frederick and Shifrer (2018) illustrate that racial minorities, including Black people, often receive more denouncing diagnoses and interventions, while less stigmatizing disability labels have been established to defend racial and class honor. For instance, the learning disability label was first created as a means for white, middle-class parents to defend their children's underperformance (Hart & Lindsay, 2024). Erevelles (2019) recommended decolonizing education by changing the traditional ways of teaching, learning, and administering education. This concept is about promoting counter and oppositional voices, knowledge, and histories and focusing on the lived experiences of students to accommodate their needs. Black scholars are encouraged to come up with techniques to continuously decolonize the education system. However, they face the challenge of Black education, demanding they become a distinctive voice in speaking and using their scholarship in youth education (Erevelles, 2019).

References

Alcoff, L. M. (2006). *Visible identities: Race, gender, and the self*. Oxford University Press.

Anderson, E. (2023). Moving the needle on ableism: From higher education access to inclusion. *Critical Perspectives in Education & Policy*, 1(1), 54–64.

Back, L. T., Keys, C. B., McMahon, S. D., & O'Neill, K. (2016). How we label students with disabilities: A framework of language use in an urban school district in the United States. *Disability Studies Quarterly*, 36(4).

Bauman, Z. (2004). *Identity: Conversations with Benedetto Vecchi*. Polity Press.

Butler, J. (1993). *Bodies that matter: On the discursive limits of "sex."* Routledge.

Butler, J. (2004). *Undoing gender*. Routledge.

Cameron, E. S., & Jefferies, K. (2021). Anti-Black racism in Canadian education: A call to action to support the next generation. *Healthy Populations Journal, 1*(1), 11–16. https://doi.org/10.15273/hpj.v1i1.10587.

Césaire, A. (1972). *Discourse on colonialism*. Trans. J. Pinkham. Monthly Review Press.

Crenshaw, K. (1989). Demarginalizing the intersection of race and sex: A black feminist critique of antidiscrimination doctrine, feminist theory and antiracist politics. *University of Chicago Legal Forum, 140*, 139–167.

Davis, L. J. (2020). Visualizing the disabled body: The classical nude and the fragmented torso. In *The Body* (pp. 167–181). Routledge.

Demetriou, K., & Symeonidou, S. (2021). Stamped allegories of disability: Representations of the disabled body on postage stamps. *Disability & Society*, 1–26.

Dei, G. J. (2017). [Re]framing blackness and black solidarities through anti-colonial and decolonial prisms: An introduction. *Reframing Blackness and Black Solidarities through Anti-Colonial and Decolonial Prisms*, 1–30. https://doi.org/10.1007/978-3-319-53079-6_1.

Du Bois, W. E. B. (1903). *The souls of black folk: Essays and sketches*. Chicago, IL: AC McClurg & Company.

Ellison, R. (1952). *Invisible man*. Random House.

Erevelles, N. (2019). "Scenes of subjection" in public education: Thinking intersectionally as if disability matters. *Educational Studies, 55*(6), 592–605. https://doi.org/10.1080/00131946.2019.1687481.

Erevelles, N., & Minear, A. (2010). Unspeakable offences: Untangling race and disability in discourses of intersectionality. *Journal of Literary Cultural & Disability Studies, 4*(2), 127–146.

Fanon, F. (1967). *Black skin, white masks*. Trans. Charles Lam Markmann. Grove Press.

Ferri, B. A., & Connor, D. J. (2006). Challenging normalcy: Dis/ability, race, and the normalized classroom. In *Reading resistance: Discourses of exclusion in desegregation and inclusion debates* (pp. 127–143). Peter Lang.

Folb, N. (2013). Chapter 14: How thinking against the grain teaches you to love what school hates. In *Youth: Responding to Lives*: Sense Publishers.

Foucault, M. (1988). *Technologies of the self: A seminar with Michel Foucault*. University of Massachusetts Press.

Foucault, M. (1995). *Discipline and punish: The birth of the prison*. Trans. Alan Sheridan. Random House.

Frederick, A., & Shifrer, D. (2018). Race and disability: From analogy to intersectionality. *Sociology of Race and Ethnicity, 5*(2), 200–214. https://doi.org/10.1177/2332649218783480.

Fuligni, A. J. (2007). *Contesting stereotypes and creating identities: Social categories, social identities, and educational participation*. Russell Sage Foundation.

Galinsky, A. D., Hugenberg, K., Groom, C., & Bodenhausen, G. V. (2003). The reappropriation of stigmatizing labels: Implications for social identity. In *Identity issues in groups* (Vol. 5, pp. 221–256). Emerald Group Publishing Limited.

Garland-Thomson, R. (1997). *Extraordinary bodies: Figuring physical disability in American culture and literature*. Columbia University Press.

Garland-Thomson, R. (2002). Integrating disability, transforming feminist theory. *NWSA Journal, 14*(3), 1–32.

Goffman, E. (1963). *Stigma: Notes on the management of a spoiled identity*. Penguin Books.

Goffman, E. (1967). *Interaction ritual: Essays on face-to-face behavior*. Anchor Books.

Grant, T., & An, M. R. P. (2021). *It's not about success, it's about access': narratives of postsecondary students labelled with invisible intellectual disabilities seeking accommodations*, Master of Social Work major research paper, Ryerson University, Canada.

Grosz, E. (2009). *The body as inscriptive surface. Volatile bodies: Towards a corporeal feminism*. Allen & Unwin.

Hart, C. M. D., & Lindsay, C. A. (2024). Teacher-student race match and identification for discretionary educational services. *American Educational Research Journal, 61*(3), 474–507. https://doi.org/10.3102/00028312241229413.

hooks, b. (1990). Marginality as a site of resistance. *Out There: Marginalization and contemporary cultures, 4*, 341–343.

Iannacci, L., & Graham, B. (2010). Mind the gap: Destabilizing dominant discourses and beliefs about learning disabilities in a Bachelor of Education program. *Alberta Journal of Educational Research, 56*(3).

Jackson, D. (2022). Making sense of Black Students' figured worlds of race, racism, anti-blackness, and blackness. *Research in the Teaching of English, 57*(1), 43–66. https://www.academia.edu/download/99686623/Making_Sense_of_Black_Students_Figured_Worlds_of_Race_Racism_Anti_Blackness_and_Blackness.pdf.

Jamil, U. (2022). Racial politics and the Postracial University. *Puncta, 5*(4), 88–105. https://doi.org/10.5399/PJCP.v5i4.6.

Jarman, M. (2012). Dismembering the lynch mob: Intersecting narratives of disability, race and sexual menace. In R. McRuer & A. Mollow (Eds.), *Sex and disability* (pp. 89–107). Duke University Press.

Mayor, C. (2023). *Trauma as white property and the erasure of Black victims: The critical trauma, anti-Black racism, and whiteness (CAW)*, Theoretical Framework.

Malacrida, C. (2016). *A special hell: Institutional life in Alberta's eugenic years*. University of Toronto Press.

Meekosha, H. (2006). What the hell are you? An intercategorical analysis of race, ethnicity, gender and disability in the Australian body politic. *Scandinavian Journal of Disability Research, 8*(2–3), 161–176.

Michalko, R. (1998). *The mystery of the eye and the shadow of blindness*. University of Toronto Press.

Michalko, R., & Titchkosky, T. (2024). Blindness and dyslexia in the movements of everyday life in Toronto. In *Placing disability: Personal essays of embodied geography* (pp. 85–93). Cham: Springer International Publishing.

Mintz, S. B., & Fraser, G. (2024). *Placing disability: Personal essays of embodied geography*. Springer Nature.

Pickens, T. A. (2017). Blue Blackness, black blueness: Making sense of blackness and disability. *African American Review, 50*(2), 93–103. https://doi.org/10.1353/afa.2017.0015.

Pickens, T. A. (2021). Blackness and disability: The Remix. *CLA Journal, 64*(1), 3–10.

Pierre, J. (2012). *The predicament of blackness.* https://doi.org/10.7208/chicago/9780226923048.001.0001.

Sagar, S., Freer, J. R., Ornstein, T., & Miller, C. J. (2024). Equal Access? Comparing Accommodation and Treatment Experiences of Racialized University Students with Attention Problems and Their White Peers. *Journal of Critical Race, Ingenuity and Decolonization, 1*(1), 40–58. https://ojs.uwindsor.ca/index.php/jcrid/issue/download/748/234#page=42.

Schechner, R. (2006). What is performance? In *Performance Studies: An introduction* (pp. 28–31).Routledge.

Smith, D. L. (1982). Social meanings versus the psychiatric concept of mental illness. *Journal of the National Medical Association, 74*(9), 917.

Titchkosky, T. (2007). *Reading and writing disability differently: The textured life of embodiment.* University of Toronto Press.

Titchkosky, T., & Michalko, R. (2009). *Rethinking normalcy: A disability studies reader.* Canadian Scholars' Press.

Trammell, J. (2009). Red-shirting college students with disabilities. *Learning Assistance Review, 14*(2), 21–31.

Toutain, C. (2019). Barriers to accommodations for students with disabilities in higher education: A literature review. *Journal of Postsecondary Education and Disability, 32*(3), 297–310.

Walcott, R. (1996). *Performing the postmodern: Black Atlantic rap and identity in North America* [Unpunished doctoral study]. University of Toronto.

Part II

The Bureaucratic Education System

In mid-December 2017, while working on my doctoral research project in the Office of Disability Studies Research, I was visited by the department chair. She requested that we speak privately. She informed me that she had been told that I had been spending more hours in the department than would be considered normal and thought it was possible that I was living in the office.

On the face of it, this would be a reasonable discussion to have with a researcher who was spending too much time in the office because they were deeply involved in academic research; however, there was no evidence that I had been using the office as living quarters. The only evidence that the office was being used for anything other than work was the length of time I spent in the space.

Rather than approaching me to determine if I had become overly involved in my academic projects, she sought to question whether I was misusing the office for my own purposes. As a person with a disability who lacked accommodations and required the use of assistive technology that was only available in the office, working long hours in the office, sometimes until 3:00 a.m., was a necessity. This confrontation and questioning was an example of the microaggressions that engaged Black and disabled scholars' experience. A scholar's efforts to overcome the lack of accommodations, in a situation where students with disabilities have too little access to resources, are met by questions regarding misuse of facilities. The lack of adequate accommodation is neither questioned nor even acknowledged. In this instance, the department chair was treating *me*, a Black student with a disability in the fifth year of study without funding, as a problem.

During the conversation, I informed the department chair about the lack of resources and that I was in my fifth year without funding and expected to complete my study in the same timeframe as non-disabled students. I explained that I required the resources in the office and that the office is a space that I had the right to occupy; however, the department chair sought to challenge my right to use the space as needed. She asked whether I had the assistive software needed to work on the project at home and, despite the lack of evidence and provision of a reasonable explanation, continued to pursue the idea that the office was being used as living quarters.

As a student with a disability, the department chair's continued challenges made it increasingly evident that her interest was in blocking my access to the accommodations that I required and that she was employing the policies and procedures of the university to do so. She inquired into how staff and security could know whether I was sleeping in my office if the office door was locked. I was then informed that I retained the privilege of using the office; however, I could only use it if sitting at my desk. I did not have the privilege of using the couch to lie on and, in fact, it would be removed from the office. I asked why she was keen to remove the couch from the Disability Studies Research office and she replied that "it is her job as the chair to protect the department." The removal of a couch from an office where disabled staff work and research about disability is performed, and where therefore, disabled, as well as non-disabled students, may be present, exemplifies a lack of effort to accommodate students who have different needs.

From this point forward, staff and security in the department behaved in a way that made me feel unwelcome in a department where I had served over seven years as a researcher for both my MEd and

PhD—and where I was continuing research on the topic of the marginalization of Black students with disabilities. A student caucus meeting was called to discuss the incident. When I asked the department chair to confirm that I was not allowed to study in my research office, she apologized for her "white privilege" and stated that she would "reflect on her actions."

Nevertheless, the chair continued to have informal, highly inappropriate, and anti-Black conversations with faculty and staff about my living status. Through January to April, when working late, a security guard would knock loudly on the office door. The knocking was disturbing and contributed to my anxiety, especially at night. When using the ground floor cafeteria, security would watch me closely and took notes when they saw me.

This came to a head on April 5, 2018, when I was carded by security and informed that because of a change in department policy, I would need to leave my office. They said that I did not have the privilege of working in my office past midnight. Thus, the staff used the bureaucracy of the school to prevent me from working diligently on my research project and instead forced me out of my office by midnight.

This barrier shows how racism and ableism in the university system still operate through bureaucratic measures to prevent students who require special accommodations from freely accessing office space needed to complete projects. Access to that space would facilitate a timely—according to the university's schedule—completion of the project. The university was not ready to either give me the time I needed to complete the project according to their deadline or allow me the privilege of using the technologies that I required and did not have access to at home. Substantial barriers arose from this lack of accommodations, contributing to the difficulties I experienced in the learning environment, imposed on me by the department chair's supposed security measures but actual fear that a Black student with a disability, working on research about the difficulties of Black disabled students, using office space to sleep. Overall, this traumatic series of events created artificial barriers to the learning experience; barriers that never needed to be created to begin with.

Chapter 4

Paradoxical Power

Solórzano et al. (2000) suggest that, at its base, racism is "a system of ignorance, exploitation, and power used to oppress" or "the belief in the inherent superiority of one race over all others and thereby the right to dominance" (p. 61). They suggest race has three key elements: (1) one group believes itself to be superior, (2) the group that believes itself to be superior has the power to carry out the racist behavior, and (3) racism affects multiple racial and ethnic groups (p. 61).

A fundamental inherent quality of racism is power and the power to oppress, assert, and act upon the beliefs of racial superiority (Wynter, 2003). The implication is that without this inherent power, there is no racism. In my interviews with Black disabled students at the University of Toronto, there is a continual citing of the power held by the administration of the university, Accessibility Services, and the professors and teaching assistants.

For example, Saga, a first-year undergraduate student, noted, "I think of the term 'disability' as being 'ableist' and another convenient way of categorizing and stigmatizing individuals based on their different learning needs." At the same time, Paige, a second-year master's student, stated that she had to avoid several barriers "while I was going through my university experience—not allowing them to block me or to stop me from, you know, experiencing or attaining what it was that I wanted to attain. Ignoring some of the stigmas, some of the snobbery that existed." Reflecting on past experience, David, a fourth-year undergraduate student, paraphrased a conversation with a professor who said he would not need to meet to discuss performance in the classroom and that "this stigma can also inform my identity and academic achievement."

The participants' experiences of marginality and stigma are important in considering the theoretical history of the self as a social and cultural production and its political and social justice implications. For example, Denise (2029), a second-year master's student, further stated:

> During a class meeting with one of my professors, he asked me if I was born in Canada because he detected an accent, and I said, "No, I was born in Jamaica." The professor's face was flushed. He asked me if I believed this was the right course for me. He further asked me whether I could speak English properly and how I got into the University of Toronto. I had to tell him that even though many Jamaicans speak broken English, they also speak proper English.

In terms of the hierarchy of the institution, the students are near the bottom of the power structure. In several instances, the students complained about racist remarks or insensitivities on the part of professors, but they avoided taking any action, citing the futility of the efforts against the power structure of the institution. In specific instances, discussed later, blatantly racist remarks are excused, with administrators accusing students of being "over-sensitive" or telling them to work it out with the professor.

The power of the university is foundational; the admissions department decides who can attend, the department's set the course and degree requirements, and Accessibility Services determines the eligibility of and accommodations for disabled students. But these powers are not exercised in a vacuum; they do have to answer to the provincial government that establishes the legislative requirements for academic accommodations as prescribed by Ontario's Human Rights

Commission and the Accessibility for Ontarians with Disabilities Act (AODA, 2023).

The stated goal of these laws and practices with regard to disabilities is to provide a "barrier free and accessible University of Toronto environment to all disabled students (AODA, 2023)." However, the university does have the latitude to decide how to comply with and structure what students must do to qualify for services or admission. Inside the bureaucracy, the subject can be lost and, as observed by many, useful service to the bureaucracy supersedes service to the individual student requiring services or accommodations. Titchkosky's (2011) insights, particularly with regard to the University of Toronto, provides a valuable backdrop for the framework of discursive bureaucratic policies and practices. It is important to work with a guiding discursive framework to understand the experiences of Black disabled students in this university by questioning the bureaucratic ordering of accommodation for those with learning differences (Titchkosky, 2011, p. 12). Sociologists have defined bureaucracy as a system of power in which the hierarchical and regularized structure of the institution governs itself and has control over others (Titchkosky, 2011; Weber et al., 1947). According to Titchkosky (2011), "These procedures are usually put into text[s] that [enforce] rules and regulations which are implemented by an office in a supposedly predictable fashion" (p. 8).

The power of the university is great, and the ability of the aggrieved student to combat racism and ableism is limited, at best, and generally viewed as inconsequential. It is therefore understandable why, when confronted by the institutional racism, many of the students stated: "Just give me my degree and let me leave." In this, we see that the student does not feel engaged in transformation and only sees the benefits of the transaction that comes from the effort expended to gain the degree, not the personal development that came with it.

Education can be perceived as an institution that helps reproduce the status quo—inequity. For Black disabled students, the education system can have a negative influence on their self-worth and identity because of the normative structures of education, including academic accommodation practices and policy, which privilege the expected student—a middle-to-upper class able-bodied white student (Dolmage,

2017; Douglas & Martino, 2020; Garland-Thomson, 1997; Goodley, 2014; Titchkosky; 2003). For students with disabilities, the classroom experience today involves the construction of normalcy and some placement in relation to it, be it one of marginalization or conformity. Wotherspoon (2014) notes that educational inclusion for students is frequently contingent upon those students accepting and emulating the standards of physical and social normalcy privileged by social institutions.

Disability and Power

Disability is often thought of in terms of what it is not. That is, it is compared to a concept of "normalcy" that somehow portrays everything else as insufficient (Titchkosky & Michalko, 2009, p. 2). Disability thus often suffers from a portrayal and categorization as a personal tragedy. Bell (2003) relates how oftentimes people who are identified as disabled are never given the choice to define themselves in terms other than ones of tragedy. Sandahl (2004) poignantly describes how, in a theatrical adaptation that describes real life experiences, the categorization of a man as both Black and blind (disabled) is problematic for the society around him as it creates confusion about which "non-normal" identity category he belongs to. It is in this context that society deals with disabled individuals. Disabled people are often viewed as a personal problem, as burdensome to society (Titchkosky & Michalko, 2009, p. 106), simply because they often cannot perform the same tasks under the same conditions as "normal" people (Taylor, 2011, p. 200).

Fanon (1967) illustrates that the marginalized subject, unable to speak or exist in a culturally "normal" way, is given an "inferiority complex" that can debilitate any hope of resistance or participation (p. 18). That is, if one accepts the notion that their identity is spoken through the language of the dominant social culture, then they may give up their ability to resist and to reclaim a more meaning identity. This results in the marginalized person always negotiating and being aware of the power of these discourses in an effort to find a way to articulate and embody an identity that is not completely determined by the powers that be. The dialectic of Blackness, disability, and normalized identity becomes perhaps even more complex in this case because more than one identity can resist the "normal."

According to McKittrick (2013), the "interlocking workings of human worth, race, and space" demonstrate "the ways the uninhabitable still holds currency in the present and continues to organize contemporary geographic arrangements" (p. 6). Additionally, interlocking identities and oppressions align with the experience of Black disabled students (Collins, 1990). For example, some have called for the reconceptualization of Blackness, class, gender, and other marginalized identities as participating in an "interlocking system of oppression" such as power (Collins, 1990, p. 536). In this chapter, the concept of "interlocking" is foundational in exposing the similarities in how categories of identity are normalized by dominant institutional powers. To be sure, there needs to be some nuance in such an analysis so as not to conflate different representations and categories of identities.

By considering Black identity in a larger sense of social and political contestation, one can productively map some of these issues onto the intersections of Blackness and disability within the educational system (Linton, 1998; Schalk, 2022). The production of social knowledge and identity is therefore influenced greatly by how racial categories are produced, reified, and shaped. It can be influenced by much of the thinking that seeks to understand the potential for identity-based resistance to take back some of the categories and definitions that have become operative in the system (Linton, 1998).

The power of institutional oppression to define the selves and bodies of Black students with disabilities is as extensive as was the power of colonial masters. As one medical authority observes, with regard to the medicalization of deviant behaviors:

> Defining deviant behavior as a medical problem allows certain things to be done that could not be otherwise considered; for example, the body may be cut open or psychoactive medications given. This treatment can be a form of social control. (Conrad, 1975, pp. 18–19)

Conrad's (1975) statement illustrates the value of considering how the social construction of the disabled self is manifested. Where oppressive social forces now veil their discursive practices with regard to Blackness, they are often still open with regard to the power they exercise over the bodies and selves of students with disabilities and their interests in promoting "social control." Conrad (1992) refers to Foucault's (1978) concept of "medical surveillance," which means that certain disabilities are viewed through a "medical gaze" that gives legitimacy to the one doing the viewing (Conrad, 1992, p. 216). This becomes a form of social and ideological control that comes to define the identities of the subjects in question. Disability is rarely imagined as a way of being—instead, it is something that affects being.

Understanding disability as a social construction, Taylor (2011) strikingly demonstrates how the disabled person is constructed by medical and institutional power as being "abnormal" and "intolerable." Indeed, Taylor underlines this point when she describes the "medical and scientific colonization [of] the disabled body" (p. 194). Thus, we should be very suspicious about the enforcement of normalized controls on identity, and Conrad's (1992, 2011) work in this regard is conversant with Foucault's critique of institutional powers that try to determine one's subjectivity. Essentially, institutions are enforcing on the disabled a set of constraints that define the nature of their disability. Just as there are constraints, the prognosis of what the disability means is predetermined and contributes to the perception of the disabled as limited in their activity.

As Titchkosky and Michalko (2009) argue:

> Disability brings normalcy into view and allows for the possibility of wondering how normalcy came about or how it was constructed in the first place. No one "normally" thinks of "normalcy." Everyone does, however, typically take normalcy for granted, thus rarely disturbing its implicit claim as being the good life and the only life worth living …. Disability … allows for the possibility of critically interrogating this claim. (pp. 6–7)

The implications of this argument are significant, for they speak not only of disabilities in our education institutions but also to the underlying taken-for-granted assumptions about what/who is valuable and what/who is not in our social environments. Within the university context, the process of obscuring the origins of normalcy and disability enable both to be taken as natural or fixed "givens." Disability and the "location" of the barriers to an individual's achievement in their body serve to obscure the arbitrary foundation of privilege among the dominant elite.

As Ferri and Connor (2006) observe, because barriers are assumed to be inherent within the individual, as opposed to structural or external, the theme of overcoming obscures the privilege enjoyed by the dominant group. As this privilege is obscured, the dominant group is positioned as deserving of success rather than specially advantaged by virtue of their social positioning.

Thus, by constructing disabilities as deviant and rooted in bodily impairment subject to "fixing," educational settings for social reproduction serve a useful role for social and political elites in obscuring the arbitrary basis of their power with the assumption that it—like disability—is a natural given in our society that can be taken for granted. Toward this end, educational institutions "need" disability to be a natural impairment of individuals' bodies, with the barriers to their aspirations being inherent in their bodies as well. In obscuring the cultural foundations of disability, these institutions also obscure the cultural foundations of power and wealth.

The notion of the intersectional is a useful tool through which to rethink how the lines of identity have been drawn, but it is also valuable in using critical Black studies to deconstruct some of the same categorical or identity issues at work in the policing of Black disabled students in the educational system. By "policing," I refer to Foucault's (1978) critique of how institutions, such as the medical clinic, enforce disciplined discourses of understanding as a compelling way of thinking about how the embodied person becomes subject to various limiting definitions.

However, Foucault focused attention on how medicalization and institutional power disciplines and controls the human body. Though it remains influential with some parts of the medical and scientific establishment, gradually, the medical model gave way to a social model of disability that conceptualizes disability as a social construct developed from the ideological and discursive practices of a society. According to the social model of disability, a visually impaired person is not disabled because they cannot see, they are disabled because the education system is designed by able-bodied people for seeing people and includes many things that are inaccessible to non-seeing people (Kuusisto, 2018, p. 4; see also Finkelstein, 2007; Oliver, 1996; Shakespeare, 2002). Given the fundamental insight of the social model of disability—that the concept of "disability" refers not to a physiological state so much as to a social construction—we can understand how disability is represented in our contemporary mediated culture in North America. I argue that this representation has "reality" in much the same way that racist representations of racialized people have "reality" in a mediated mass culture, with both being social constructions that validate and support systemic discrimination against particular groups.

For example, as hooks (1992) notes, the production of meaning about identity within popular culture is involved in a hegemonic process. She argues that Black identity is defined in the mass media as being self-consciously subordinate to white male identity:

> They [Black people] are represented in this manner by white cultural productions, particularly in television, film, and advertising. The colonizing culture's manipulation of representation is necessary for the maintenance of white-supremacist capitalist patriarchy. (p. 105)

In hooks' view, Black identity is created by white dominated popular culture through the production of meaning about Black bodies. While these meanings, and the identities they frame, can often be completely absurd and divorced from reality, this qualification is insignificant in comparison with the need for the corporate producers of popular culture to project stabilizing, hegemonic discourses. A popular cultural artifact has the potential to illustrate how the creation of meaning about bodies can be critically hegemonic with respect to larger societal concerns about identity.

McKittrick (2000), who discusses the issue of the body of the Black woman, reviews the narrative of poet and author Marlene Philip, discussing how she had influenced the nature of the social construction of the Black woman's body and how subjectivities and dominant narratives had a role in the way the body was understood and how it is that Black womanhood is unique. This critical analysis is distinct from the investigation of other categorizes Blackness intersects with. In this analysis, the woman's body is constructed as being different from the man's. There are limitations in the scope of the capabilities of women but also ways for women to contribute to society. Women are understood to offer something crucial that men cannot. This differs from disability, which is understood as something that must be overcome. The woman is not expected to overcome her difference in physical attributes. They are needed.

As this is the case, while sexism persists, the experience of disability is unique from sexism—while both women and the disabled are considered to be creating a dependency, the extent to which this happens is much different among women than among men.

Identity, in this more social sense, becomes the complex understanding of who we are. Titchkosky (2000) discusses how intersectional marginalization of different elements of identity contribute to the condition of individuals that are poor, Black, or disabled. She describes how people at this intersection are perceived of as naturally vulnerable, and the social and economic differences people at this intersection experience can be excused as the inevitable result of being Black and disabled. Factors such as the wage gap, unemployment, and the lack of empowerment experienced by Black and disabled people are therefore constructed as based on the disparity between the opportunities for people from their social background and the limited abilities to perform tasks among the disabled. Little consideration is given to how social differences are a consequence of a recursive system that holds back people who are disabled.

Just as Black and disabled people are considered vulnerable, so too are "normal" people strong. In this view, Black and disabled people are dependent on the non-disabled and the non-racialized (i.e., white) people for social and economic opportunity and development. By normalizing this idea of their "vulnerability," we also normalize the marginality that Black disabled individuals experience. Students are put in a position where social institutions must accommodate them, and the administrators must create policies enforcing different treatment for the disabled based on the different nature of their capabilities.

Ultimately, we have approached the discussion of how disability and Blackness are understood, and of the elements of identity and the social and economic aspects of life that come with them, from an understanding of how the impairments and diverse abilities contribute to different ways of life.

Titchkosky (2000) suggests that disability is a social construct that enacts stigmatization, making normalcy distinguishable for the people understood to "belong" to the university (p. 204). Disability identification, in this sense, can support racism by contributing to the marginalization of Black students with disabilities. Thus, visual signifiers of marginalization—Blackness, disability, and gender—function as normative mechanisms to enact not only lowered expectations but also other forms of oppression. Wynter (1994) notes that the struggles with Blackness, disability, gender, and class are bound up in a history of oppression that has been propagated by colonization and imperialism. That is, we can take note of the differences in racialized embodiment without resorting to those more pernicious ideas about physiological differences per se.

In this way, defining disability as marginal to the ordinary goings-on of university life limits some people while allowing the taken-for-granted members to use other people's marginalization to validate the dominant normative state of university life and work. This presents the problem of how to define what disabled identity is or how it can be phrased. Butler (1993) argues that the post-modern critique leads to a more productive understanding of gender, identity, and race (Blackness) in terms of how one conforms to these categories. Their emphasis is on the body and identity insofar as it is inscribed with ideas and definitions that are often part of a dominant discourse.

In the same way, Foucault (1978) suggests that post-modern thought generally operates by interrogating the discourses that are embedded in educational institutions and practices. That is, if identity cannot be ascribed to any stable categories of being, then it must be a constructed product of society and political discourses. This implies that the notion of normalcy is a power construct that shapes not only how we think about our own identities but also the assumptions we make about others' identities (Titchkosky & Michalko, 2009).

Defining Black disabled students through "abnormality" is degrading because it suggests that a "normal" life is the only one worth living (Titchkosky & Michalko, 2009, p. 4)—and maybe the only one worth imagining. And this approach is taken by many administrative personnel in universities and in other official institutions such as the Canadian government (Titchkosky & Michalko, 2009, p. 5). As a result of this approach, some people in power believe that accommodations afford the disabled students an easier test environment, giving them an advantage over other members of the class. David had this experience when a professor refused to meet with him regarding a grade:

> I received a low grade on one of my assignments, which I worked very hard on and thought I should've gotten a higher grade. I asked the professor if it was possible for me to meet with him to discuss my grade. He told me that there is no need for that because students with disabilities should be given the same exam time as non-disability students and as far as he is concerned, I have an advantage over my course-mates.

Many of the students also strongly disagreed with being labeled disabled even though they receive assistance from Accessibility Services because of a learning disorder; for these students, they just learn differently and require alternate means or a different environment for testing to compete with other mainstream students.

This sentiment was expressed most vociferously by Saga, when he boldly declared: "I ain't disabled, [I have] different learning needs." Kimberly (2019) a Second year Masters Humanities and Social Sciences also preferred to see herself as having different learning "needs":

> I will not agree to be called disabled—I will not label myself as a Black disabled student. I choose not to label myself as disabled. I do accept that I'm a Black student in the social context. The idea of being a disabled student—I do not agree with the term because I feel that everyone's learning needs or learning issues are unique to him or her. So when they assess services or they have learning issues in the school, they may be approached in a different context and have different experiences.

She can accept the "social context" of being a Black student as a statement of fact, but avoiding the term disabled qualified her learning experience as different but not due to an individual impairment. The general appraisal by those interviewed was that learning disabilities, as classified by Accessibility Services, do not constitute a true disability; for many, "disabled" refers to a physical impairment. For example, Christine said:

> I have a hard time dealing with what they call [being a] disabled student. I didn't like it. I didn't consider myself disabled because my granddad is blind. He's dead now but he was blind. And so, when I thought of disability, I thought of him. I thought of "disabled" as someone who is physically impaired.

This sentiment is echoed in the responses from students who indicated they have physical impairments. In the case of Folake, a second-year graduate student in the humanities and social sciences who suffers from chronic back pain, she noted that her disability is invisible, which means she struggles with it all the more. She added that she fears her professors and accessibility advisors will not believe her when she voices her extreme discomfort and often feels the need to just tolerate the pain so as to not raise undue scrutiny or criticism:

> My disability is invisible, a chronic back pain. I always have this consciousness of fear that if I tell my professors or accessibility advisors that I wasn't feeling well, and I wasn't able to do an exam or complete an assignment on time they would not believe me. However, if I experience pain during class time, I still forced myself to school. I am afraid that my professors would think that I am faking my illnesses.

From this perspective, the cultural context of Blackness, disability, class, and gender played a role in the perceptions of many of these students (Collins, 1990, p. 540), as when Folake experienced accommodation as vulnerability. Drawing on Black feminist thought, one can identify the need to resist domination by social institutions, such as universities (Collins, 1990, p. 541).

This particular theory is captured in Folake's insight regarding the need to "deal" with the professors, accessibility advisors, and others who are supposed to help her with her disability but often made her feel that she needed to prove or justify that she was entitled to the services and not looking to "game" the system. Despite Folake's apprehension about dealing with these university services, she continued to do so because she understood that pursuing these services not only ensured she got the assistance she was entitled to but was also a way to resist the institutional barriers that she believed were placed in those settings.

Nevertheless, some of the students facing learning challenges did not voice objections to the "disabled" label. Several of the students even embraced their disability. They did not view their disability as a disadvantage or insurmountable challenge, rather it was an integral part of their identity and part of their student experience at the University of Toronto. Barry is a first-year undergraduate arts and sciences student who took pride in accepting the label placed on him:

> I am proud to be a Black disabled man. But being Black and disabled is very challenging for me in the university. I've been asked many times by my peers how did I get into to such an elite university and if I have what it takes to succeed in it.

This sense of pride and idea of accepting the challenge was a reoccurring theme in several interviews. Paige phrased the sentiment succinctly by simply stating, "I've learned to ignore certain aspects of how I'm treated, and what to some people it means to be labeled disabled. But that's me! Because that's my personality!"

Still, many students were hesitant, reluctant, defiant, or ambivalent in making a declaration that they were disabled. Nonetheless, all were in agreement that disability self-identification was necessary if one were to qualify for Accessibility Services accommodations. This identification was universally accepted as an indispensable aspect of their university experience, yet it presented many difficulties. The students all indicated that they needed the accommodations and support associated with embracing this label for adaptive and/or financial reasons, despite the accompanying stigma and administrative entanglements. Nearly all students had lived with a disability for their entire lives, some learned to live with it on their own and spent several years at university without assistance, and many learned to hide their disability from their peers to avoid marginalization. Though some embraced their disability, many reluctantly accepted the label, and all acknowledged that others perceived this label as an unflattering way to describe their identity.

Titchkosky and Michalko (2009) state that studying disability is only possible if researchers (and ultimately society) release their hold on the concept of normalcy and approach the research from a more pluralistic view of human experience (p. 11). Titchkosky (2007) suggests that disability is an opportunity to evaluate how identities are constructed and how we might otherwise construct meaning in the relations between people (p. 16). The idea that the so-called dependency of disabled students on others is a burden on the system fails to recognize the interconnectedness of society and how dependent we all are on each other. In actuality, disabled students' lives are made difficult by the existence of systems and tools that are constructed for the non-disabled population (Taylor, 2011, p. 201). By adhering to a model of normalcy and seeing accommodation of disabled individuals as an "extra" step, rather than recognizing a plurality of experiences, society in effect creates disability (Shakespeare & Watson, 2002, p. 11). Or, as Oliver (1996) said:

> In our view, it is society which disables physically impaired people. Disability is something imposed on top of our impairments by the way we are unnecessarily isolated and excluded from full participation in society. Disabled people are therefore an oppressed group in society. (p. 22)

Indeed, the power of institutional oppression to define the selves and bodies of people with disabilities is effectively an absolute power.

As noted earlier, the social model of disability suggests that it is society that renders disabled people as such by not organizing itself to include them (Shakespeare & Watson, 2002, pp. 9–12). Thinking about this differently, Shakespeare (2002), in one of his earlier discussions of how the social model of disability differs from other political framings of disability, observes how perceptions of disability in North America have clear analogies with the civil rights struggle, which has been significant in transforming our understanding of race and culture. Shakespeare observes, "The North American approach has mainly developed the notion of people with disabilities as a minority group, within the traditions of US political thought" (p. 4). Shakespeare makes a case for disability theorists—particularly those in the United Kingdom—to consider a revision of the social model of disability, which had become the orthodox critical model for understanding disability in the academic context.

The culture of disability is influenced by the way economics, society, and policy impact the disabled person, along with their recursive impact back on policy, economics, and society. Many researchers approach disability from the perspective that the social phenomenon has marginalized the disabled person to the point of disempowerment as successful contributors to the world. The experience of disability is unique in that disabled students understand themselves as "problems" that must be solved. Titchkosky (2000) discusses how scholars have described disability in the past, building their understanding of disability on information from people who have had experience with the disabled, not people who are themselves disabled. Titchkosky (2007) raises an important point in noting that disability, and other identity categories, do not exist in isolation but always as part of an enactment between people. These categories are not simply individual consciousnesses, they are an interaction between different consciousnesses (p. 23). Thus, it is only in the realization of the inequities built into these categories that the process of "disidentification" can take place (Muñoz, 1999).

It is important to consider the cultural role of the Black disabled person in societies where the disabled are considered to have a problem that requires solving. These disabled people *are* problems whose existence would require those who are not disabled to solve them. But Black or disabled people are *not* problems and should not be viewed through a paternalistic lens. That leads to ableist and racist policies that place them in a position where they depend on able-bodied, white people "fixing" them or designing a path through which they must live their lives. This is not a socially just approach to the position of the disabled in society. It is regressive in nature because it supposes that the able-bodied (as they may be) have superior power and influence through their able-bodiedness (Goodley et al., 2019; Johnson & McRuer, 2024; Michalko, 2002).

Alongside recognizing differences and pluralities of human experience, it is also necessary to desire such pluralities, such alterities

(Titchkosky, 2007, p. 25). Simply attempting to address systemic inequity is not possible without addressing the patterns of behavior that define and "perform" social identity within society (Dei, 2022; Kannen, 2008, p. 149). Moreover, disability has been investigated from the perspective of being related to "problem people," with the idea that society must work with the disabled to overcome their troubles.

The implication of this is that the disabled bring with them flaws that must be dealt with if a disabled person is brought into a work, education, or other social institution setting. Disability is therefore a social problem that extends beyond the disabled individual and will have implications for people who remain in the social sphere of the disabled. From an administrative standpoint, this can mean specific accommodations for the disabled; however, these accommodations further support the notion of the disabled being a problem requiring solutions rather than aiding the empowerment of the disabled student.

In order for these accommodations to be respected by a bureaucratic system, they must become a part of the policy directing the system. The structure of the bureaucracy poses the problems; however, it can also function as a solution when suitable policies are designed and accepted into the system. They must support the continuation of the bureaucratic system as a productive, efficient, and effective entity. The crafting of policy that would grant the required accommodations for Black disabled students would require a clear understanding of how disabilities and Blackness are linked in the experience of Black university students.

This book sheds light on Accessibility Services, which espouses a policy of inclusion yet practices routine exclusions while paying "lip service" to respect for disabled students. The university as a bureaucracy is keen on self-preservation. Based on Weber's (1947) conceptualizations, its administrators routinely invoke policies and procedures that maintain the entrenched hierarchical structure. In so doing, they engage in practices that tend to resist meaningful or even sustainable structural change.

For instance, some students reported that they experienced racial discrimination or were treated as a problem by Accessibility Services administration when they sought accommodations from them. Thus, inequity due to disability and Blackness suggests that these laws and policies, however strong or well-meaning, are not enough without deep-seated acceptance of the need for inclusion, support services, and reasonable accommodations for students with disabilities.

The wide differences in the perception of Blackness and disability in classroom settings represent critical evidence that disability is not a physical given but a cultural construct. For Black disabled students, understanding disability in the classroom as a complex sociopolitical phenomenon opens the possibility of a more complex critical analysis of inclusion and exclusion and, ultimately, a more just and progressive pedagogy for learners and educators in the twenty-first-century classroom.

The social model of disability should be revised to conceptualize disability not only as a social mode of oppression but also as a model that incorporates issues of identity. Foucault (1978), writing on the history of sexuality, for example, reveals how the discourses that encouraged repression actually served to uphold a bourgeois order and economic system. He defines the relations between sex and power as one that has used ideas of prohibition, silence, and transgression to "discipline" or "control" bodies that fall outside the norms of society.

Gilroy (2005) asserts that Foucault's (1978) critique is not so distant from the above statements of colonial power, especially that of Fanon (1967), which exposed how domineering forces created categories of human and non-human or civilized or uncivilized to set up a system of institutions that could police these differences. Gilroy's analysis of post-colonial melancholia is directly related to post-modern critiques of institutions and cultures that attempt to "educate" subjects about what it is to be a human or what it is like to be a Black person within a more dominant culture. The concept of institutional power has been revealed in previous sections, noting that it is intrinsic to the discriminations of accommodations by Accessibility Services. As noted by one research participant, Stephanie (2019), it takes courage and determination to stand up to an institutional power that insists on complete capitulation to their requirements and submission to obtain services; worse, there is an institutional lack of respect and a racial hierarchy in accessing accommodations at Accessibility Services.

Likewise, Foucault (1995) holds that the foundation of omnipresence in a hierarchal structure resides in his theory that it is within society as a whole that power is spread to the masses. Within this construct, the power of social relationships is determined by how knowledge and techniques of control were developed by the society. Foucault defines this through his understanding of the widely dispersed collusion of social relationships that stem from institutional and cultural influence (Cahill, 2000, p. 47). For him, power is not something that can stem from any particular part of society; rather, it is an inherent part of the structure of how human beings interact with one another. Although major institutions, like the military or educational institutions, may be a part of the way power is distributed, it is social "discourse" that allows human beings to be taken into these multifaceted systems when they adhere to a particular identity. This subjective nature of power becomes part of a more personal and larger interaction between social discourses that does not emanate from any single idea.

However, Foucault does not imply that power simply comes from all directions and without a purpose; some institutions impose a non-subjective and intentional discourse that allows power to be distributed throughout society. In this manner, the essence of power arises from society as a whole, but it is also enacted from the non-subjective discourse of larger social institutions that define and enforce various norms and regulations—this is the operation of power producing its subjects.

Double Consciousness

DuBois' (1903) early writing on double consciousness is essential to my initial evaluation of the significance of Black studies on disability because one has to negotiate two different categories of identity, even though it is arguable that both remain tied to the identity of a marginalized group. As discussed in the following section, their double consciousness is witnessed by theorists of Blackness and disability as subjects negotiate multiple identities or find some ways of bridging them coherently.

This represents a significant challenge for anyone interested in critically evaluating how Black and disability studies matter in the university. They provide a strong theoretical foundation for the kinds of discussions that need to happen with respect to how one might escape the trap of seeing oneself only through the eyes of the medical authorities (e.g., biomedicine) that define the experience and the idea of being a "normal" embodied subject. The dominated spaces wherein these identities are constructed are of concern for any critic who is interested in addressing them.

I argue that one must work through some of these earlier complications of race representation to arrive at a better understanding of how these different, but sympathetic, identities can relate to each other and create a critical conversation about marginalization, normative views, and representation. Black identity, seen in this way, becomes a kind of dialectical process of existing within this representation of doubleness or hybridity (Bhabha, 1994; DuBois, 1903). It is also a psychological formulation insofar as the consciousness of the individual is shaped by both their racial identification and by the powers of the dominant culture or race that create normalized ideas of what it is to hold this identity.

In considering this point, I look at the dichotomy between identity-based resistance and the later postmodern attempts to challenge the fixities in any categories of identity representation. DuBois' (1903) concept of "double consciousness" has been influential in theorizations of race insofar as it points to a site of psychological and social contestation within the experience of Black identity. His concept of double consciousness aligns with contemporary post-colonial theorists (Gilroy, 2000; Hall, 2001) who also suggest that Black people find themselves living in-between two camps or two categories of identity and belonging. These scholars theorized that there is a dislocation of identity at times when one must negotiate different cultural ideas of identity and race that confront each other or create a feeling of hybridity, to use Bhabha's (1994) notion. The representation of Blackness is therefore a complex one that has raised issues of identity formulations as a mode of political resistance (hooks, 1992).

As hooks (1992) pointed out, theorizing Black experience remains a "difficult task" since it is often "normalized" by educational systems (p. 2). She maintains, "Many Black people are convinced that our lives are not complex, and therefore unworthy of sophisticated critical analysis" (p. 2). This view represents one of the central threads within race, theory, and the post-colonial experience of the marginalized because it asks people to consider how complexities in identity representations are constructed and influenced by hegemonic cultural norms and narratives and need to be untangled or reimagined as contested (Gilroy, 2000). Thus, hooks argues that productively resisting identity and cultural norms is "a fundamental task of Black critical thinkers ... struggling to break with the hegemonic modes of seeing, thinking that block our capacity to see ourselves oppositionally to imagine, describe, and invent ourselves in ways that are liberatory" (p. 2).

hooks' (1992) claims have productively impacted my own thinking on both Blackness and disability because they expose this notion that embodiment is connected to having a space with which to see oneself in opposition to dominant and normal representations. The liberatory impulse in these critical reflections on racial identity can be applied to the even more complicated question of how one who is marginalized both by race and disability can counteract and resist the hegemonic identity constructs that have been forced upon them.

Recognizing this tension as a key problem in how the identities of Black and disability interact and counteract normalized ideas is central to my research. It is a first step in thinking about how best to theorize the problem in the field. Strategies for resistance should be worked out carefully because there are pitfalls in the identity-based politics of resistance. In his book *The Wretched of the Earth* Fanon (1961) argues that national consciousness will be "an empty shell, a crude and fragile traversity" (p. 148). He lists what he considers the pitfalls of national consciousness. These include primitive tribalism, especially where social consciousness is achieved before real nationalism, class differences and the bourgeoisie, the people's pacification and the people's alienation from the masses, and lack of a national identity or authentic nationalism. These pitfalls are the reasons critical thinkers such as hooks and DuBois can be foundational for exposing how this double consciousness creates a "master/slave dialectic" in the mind of the oppressed (Fanon, 1963). That is, following DuBois' use of the concept of double consciousness, Fanon (1963) writes that being the "other" is connected to the notion of the world. He writes, "What parcels out the world is to begin with the fact of belonging to or not belonging to a given race, a given species" (p. 40).

The doubleness alluded to in Dubois' phrase "double consciousness" refers to the racial minorities' and the disabled people's psychological experience of having to navigate their identities in two or more various contexts. In the first context, they are innately aware of their own identity. In the second, they are also acutely aware of how they are perceived by white people in dominantly white societies. This duality or doubleness means that individuals must navigate their identities from their own lenses and the given identities stemming from the perspective of the white spectacle (Fanon, 1963). As discussed in the earlier chapter on colonialism of the mind, the colonial project had a psychological dimension in addition to the physical dimension. The colonizers imposed on the racial minorities Western and Eurocentric views on African culture depicting Black culture and race as inferior. This was done with the intention of acculturating Black communities to challenge them to abandon their long-held perceptions of their identities and adopt the Western or Eurocentric way, which was considered universal, authentic, and superior (Kgatla, 2018; Oelofsen, 2015). However, the acculturation involves a psychological process where the subjects must navigate between competing and parallel identities or narratives. Racial minorities must reconcile the perception of their self-image with the external perception propagated by the social structures and racial prejudices.

The master/slave dialectic is an inevitable consequence of double consciousness. The master/slave dialectic has its origins in the philosophical works of Georg Wilhelm Friedrich Hegel (2019), specifically *The Phenomenology of Spirit*. Dialectic simply means an investigation into the truthfulness of an opinion and rational inquiry into the metaphysical contradictions between two or more competing narratives. Hegel argues that the dialectic movement sought to examine the truthfulness of the various philosophical expositions, noting that truth is itself subjective (p. 30). The master/slave dialectic is the psychological state of the oppressed. They seek to identify what their truthful identity is, between a slave and a master. The oppressed Black minorities (enslaved) look up to the white supremacist (master) for recognition of their self-consciousness because social recognition is essential to the existence of the consciousness. However, with the master seeking to keep the slave subjugated, withholding recognition thereby keeps the slave in a state of dependence (p. 114). With time, however, the slave's consciousness broadens as they become more and more aware of their oppression, leading to a liberation and subversion of the problematic master/slave dynamic. This explains why Black racial minorities internalize the values of their oppressors, staying in a state of subjugation for some time and ultimately rising against the racist conceptions of their identities. This concept applies not only to Black racial minorities but also to disabled people in a society that is undergirded by the hegemonic ideologies of ableism.

There is an abundance of research that addresses Blackness and what it means within different institutions. Narratives from critical Black writers contribute to an in-depth understanding of Black studies because they are a voice for the experience of people who are less likely to be heard because they lack privilege in higher education. Nonetheless, scholars should inform scholarly work and enhance Black studies. After all, the scholarly system has been designed by people with privilege, without providing access for Black and disabled people. Lorde (1984) notes that "the master's tools will never dismantle the master's house" (p. 112). In this context, she means that it is necessary to work outside the confines of traditional scholarly practice when investigating Blackness because of the control non-racialized people have had on that practice.

In her work, Lorde (1984) describes women at the intersection of Blackness as being at the lowest end of the societal hierarchy; however, for those with privilege, people in this position are the most threatening. She describes the differences between Black people and other people in the population as a factor that creates strength and argues that the genuine change to the social order that they seek is a significant threat to the privileged. While the privileged will allow people without privilege to "beat him at his own game" (p. 112), Lorde reminds us that, by doing this, Black people and women continue to play the game, and this has contributed to their intersectional marginalization. Administrative regulation does not protect people who are marginalized; it continues their dependence on a system that has left them without privilege.

Lorde's (1994) narrative is important because it expresses her experience in the social hierarchy, which she perceives as a lack of access for Black women based on institutional elements. Her works are critical of popular culture and the ways it supports the system (Lorde, 1994). hooks describes the acceptance of advertising, fashion, and popular culture as designed by white people at the top of the social hierarchy as damaging to Blackness.

While Black studies and disability studies are proposed as belonging together because of the marginality of these different elements of identity, a more robust approach to the issue of academic study in the scope of Black studies is needed. Because of the nature of the social production of racial scripts and how they take on a biologically deterministic nature, Lorde (1994) suggests that a highly interdisciplinary approach to the study of Blackness that incorporates other factors, such as science, geography, and Black creative texts, would move us beyond the scope of traditional Black studies, which focuses on the arts.

Normal

The construction of "normal" is a manifestation of social and cultural power that is read and written by educational systems upon the bodies of both able people and people with disabilities. These systems sometimes harness medical authorities and other unexamined societal assumptions about both Blackness and disability. This calls into question the normative standards that are offered by the educational system or the medical authorities, which create identities based on European notions of how people are expected to fit. Disability, in this sense, is not so much a physical reality as a social construction that historically and culturally frames individuals as "different," as having an impairment, and thereby having or being a problem with and for the normal order of things, including education.

A cultural frame—like a picture frame—represents a line or means of demarcating and can be conceived of as a social limit. Disability, much like Blackness (another "mistake" of DNA replication? [Gilroy, 2000]), has historically been deployed to limit the opportunities and potential of individuals with disabilities. The concept of "normal" must therefore be questioned in terms of how it is used in education and social institutions to support restrictive conceptions of disability and racial identity (Hall, 2001).

Following from the premise that the education system continues to be a "construction site" for normalcy, I consider how Black students with disabilities, who do not reflect the privileged normative way of being, will not enjoy easy accommodations to help them with their studies, nor other successes that education is supposed to offer. Disability studies interrogates' normalcy, with scholars pointing out that "the problem is not the person with disabilities; the problem is the way that normalcy is constructed to create the problem of the disabled person" (Davis, 1995, p. 24). One of the basic principles in disability studies today is the theory that normality and disability are not references to physical realities so much as constructions defined and developed by social institutions:

> The meanings attributed to extraordinary bodies reside not in inherent physical flaws, but in social relationships in which one group is legitimated by possessing valued physical characteristics and maintains its ascendancy and self-identity by systematically imposing the role of cultural or corporeal inferiority upon others. (Garland-Thomson, 1997, p. 7)

As this passage suggests, the associated concepts of "normalcy" and "disability" are both products of social power that have historically had, as a fundamental effect, a discriminatory role in social relations. These power relations were reinforced by the cultural representations of deviance in association with Blackness and disability. Thus, Blackness and disability make an appearance as representation, and these representations have "reality" in the sense that they can determine and limit the social potential of the students upon whom they are imposed.

These representations often carry with them overtones of "deviance" that implicitly separate the objects of the gaze from the educational community surrounding them. As coded in these representations, deviance is a complex social phenomenon. Becker (1963) notes, "Social groups create deviance by making the rules whose infraction constitutes deviance and by applying these rules to particular people and labeling them as outsiders" (p. 9).

Viewed from this perspective, representations of Blackness and disability can carry with them "codes" that mark the object of the representation as distinct from the educational institutions that define the codes and the representations that carry them. This is one of the subtle ways systematic discrimination operates in social institutions, including those of higher education. This systematic discrimination is rarely overt, and so it is difficult to empirically measure its operation. Nonetheless, those who are subject to it recognize its power.

The difficulty of measuring the effect of such social representations may be one reason to value autobiographical writing as a scholarly tool. These works obviously lack statistical significance, yet they allow critics to address elusive and subtle social operations. One of the interesting features of these representations is how they depend for their power upon the social acceptance of their objectivity. For Black people, their representation in Euro-American culture has been marked for centuries by the close intertwining of racial identity and anti-Black racism with deviance.

Indeed, as scholars have noted, the construction of the default "normality" in Euro-American culture occurs not only with respect to individuals' status as non-disabled/disabled but also in terms of gender and race. For example, the "normate" in this cultural context is white, male, heterosexual, and able-bodied (Garland-Thomson, 1997, p. 8; Goodley, 2014). Similarly, Titchkosky (2003) notes:

> "Normate" is a concept that references the idea of an unmarked category of persons that are culturally regarded as "definitive human beings" ... for example: white, able-bodied, average height, white teeth, unblemished ... heterosexual, male, etc., wielding authority and power .... Normate is also made use of to bracket the taken-for-granted status of normalcy. (p. 157)

Viewed through this lens, Black disabled students do not have the chance of ever being considered "normal" since to be perceived as Black and disabled is to simultaneously be perceived as and made marginal. Educational institutions are dependent on keeping some members of the student population marginal. By keeping these students marginal, they gain a number of social, political, and economic benefits. The "normate" is defined by those with the "cultural capital" to rely on their particular bodily configurations and to define the normative human and thereby accentuate their own social and cultural authority at the expense of those classified as possessing such marginalizing features as disability.

Scholars have noted that there are clear associations between this general discriminatory process and discrimination in terms of Blackness and disability in the education system. As Garland-Thomson (1997) writes, "The non-normate status accorded disability feminizes all disabled figures" (p. 9). As this statement indicates, the construction of "normalcy" and "disability" possess clear analogies to the social processes involved in Blackness, class, and gender discrimination in our society.

Consider, for example, how the classification of students with disabilities occurs in our contemporary classrooms. In the case of students categorized under the rubric of "learning difficulties," observers have noted that "socio-economic and cultural factors interfere with the development of cognitive and language skills" (Barnes & Wade-Wooley, 2007, p. 9). Similar inadequacies are evident in the diagnostic assessment criteria and identification procedures for learners with disabilities in sciences, which has led to "the number of students identified as having a math disability [being] over-inflated" (Baptist et al., 2007, p. 14). Conversely, Foster (2007) also points to controversy over how schools disproportionately assign white students to classes for "gifted learners" and place Black students in special education programs (p. 36).

However, critical disability studies facilitate the analysis of the cultural construction of disabilities in the classroom, and we—like the characters in *The Wizard of Oz* (Fleming, 1939)—are enabled to see "behind the curtain" and interrogate otherwise hidden operations of power in our educational institutions. There is a moment in the classic *Wizard of*

Oz film when the puny wizard who has disguised himself behind the illusion of the great and powerful Oz is sniffed out by Dorothy's dog, Toto. Realizing he has been exposed, he attempts to recover his power by commanding Dorothy and her friends with the famous line: "Pay no attention to that man behind the curtain." This classic movie scene serves as a useful illustration of the complex reasons educators "need" disability in the classroom. It is through the cultural definition of deviance, in terms of cultural markers such as race, disability, gender, and class, that the medical models shape the understanding of how normalcy is enforced in our educational institutions—and ultimately in society itself.

Consequently, "normal" is one of those apparently innocuous terms that can have a devastating emotional effect upon those students who lie outside the peak of the bell curve. When a student is on the "wrong end" of the curve of normality, they are likely to be marginalized and stigmatized. In terms of socioeconomic status and physical ability, the word "normal" sets the scales for "privileged," "disadvantaged," "abled," and "disabled." Some people suggest that a suitable synonym for "normal" is "average," but with regards to education, it is often the terms "acceptable," "expected," or "standard" and the antonym "abnormal" that are at work. Additionally, conditions that lie within the majority are considered "normal (Davis, 1995, p. 35)."

Unfortunately, when discussing normalcy, abilities and even Blackness become intertwined with these terms with racist or in the most extreme cases eugenicist consequences (Davis, 1995, p. 35). Able and white students would be considered "normal," with the Black disabled students falling outside the "normal" range. When related to these terms, this discussion seems absurd; however, the experience of the students in this research relates to a different interpretation of "normal." They are experiencing university education outside normalcy. As noted above regarding Blackness, there were lower expectations of the racial minority student on the University of Toronto campus.

Folake sees things this way:

> There is also the maintenance of racist stereotypes in the university and the demonizing of Black students. If a Black student should not live up to the

university "expectations," then the entire Black student population will be ostracized. I believe our collective Blackness becomes the embodiment of these spaces. The university likes to brag about how diverse they are, but anti-Black racism is so normalized here such as in the classrooms, with my peers and administration personnel.

From this perspective, we need to move away from the nice buzzwords—diversity, inclusion, accessibility, equity. Like all buzzwords that are continually cited in the documents of political and education institutions, they lose their power to assist in creating general change in our society. According to Thomas-Long (2010), diversity in the university is a continual struggle for Black students, which is closely related to the issue of access and equity. A university may use "respect for diversity" in its Mission Statement but may, in practice, be far from actually approaching it. Instead, I assert that universities must address the hard questions of our time frankly, openly, and without silencing marginalized voices.

Speaking to the terms "normal" and "abnormal" as applied to race and ability, Saga stated:

> What is a "normal" person? Or what do we expect a disabled person to look like? Are we not human beings anyway? We're defined based on our categorization such as our Blackness, disability, gender, and sexuality surrounding the "abnormal."

Noting that because he is Black and disabled—though, as noted before, he does not consider himself disabled—he feels the university does not consider him "normal." This was a common experience with other students as well. Sarah, a second-year PhD Sciences student, spoke to that antonym of normal—"incompetent"—to observe:

> It's interesting because we assume disability means incompetency. I often say I am high-functioning, which is problematic because it means you're assuming disability means you can't be high-functioning. I think a lot of my professors had to come to terms with the idea that I was a Black female with a disability. And I was one of the highest performing students ... since I was studying sciences. It was obvious I wasn't "normal" in their eyes and that I was not supposed to be there. I would sit in the office and ask questions.

I would have professors look at me and shake their heads in front of me and give all kinds of body language to show they thought I was stupid.

This is a student who was performing at the highest levels but, due to her Blackness and disability, was considered stupid by her professors—all because of attitudes associated with the concepts of normalcy and majority. Discussing stigma in the university, Titchkosky (2015) suggests that "disability and [Blackness] are used to point out the act of dehumanization within the social political orders of the day and are also used for the ongoing accomplishment of dehumanization" (p. 6).

Most of the students indicated learning disabilities as a reason they were classified as disabled, and some indicated that they learned differently, had trouble concentrating in classroom settings, or needed a few accommodations. None of the students indicated that their learning disability was a deficit, nor that they could not function as university students; some had already earned university degrees. In other words, the concept of normalcy should not apply to a person's ability to be in the university and compete academically with other students. As I discussed in the previous section of this chapter, the bell curve is employed as a yardstick to measure the Black disabled students against their able peers and stigmatizing them as different and, in many ways, as inferior.

I claim that an ordinary perception of disability is not informed by disability studies but by unexamined conceptions of disability that conform to the normative order of society (Davis, 1995; Garland-Thomas, 1997; Titchkosky, 2000). While the differences between the two are complex, I argue that the former focuses on the individual with a disability, representing their life as a management problem, while the latter shifts critical attention on "normate" society itself and the processes of cultural production it fosters, imposing a range of cultural preconceptions about people with disabilities on both these people and the society at large. Although challenging these preconceptions can be unsettling—particularly given how pervasive and powerful these conceptions can be—this book offers the possibility of systemically disrupting oppressive social hegemonic disability-knowledge in this regard.

Discriminatory Culture

A reoccurring theme throughout the interview process was the issue of stigma and marginalization. The students reported feeling stigmatized with respect to both their identity as a racial minority, Black, and as a disabled student receiving accommodations for their disability. The university has made a long-standing claim of being a welcoming environment for racialized bodies, claiming that the strength of the student population lies with its diversity, and that diversity is an essential part of the university experience. The experiences of the students in this book do not fit the stated goals of the university with respects to diversity. The most glaring examples of this were the several instances of blatant racially disparaging comments and attitudes that went unchecked and tacitly condoned by the university.

The first example is of the "smart monkey" comments related by one of the students. Sarah shared, "In my third year [of] undergrad, I had a male professor who made a lot of problematic comments including references to smart monkeys [emphasis added] during lectures. He also said some of these things to me personally." This conduct was so prevalent with this professor that she considered taking action:

> Interviewer: Did the professor make these comments privately or in class?
> Participant: Some of them were private and some were during lectures. For example, there was a comment made by the professor about "smart monkeys." However, some students didn't have a clue that such comments are wrong, as they've never dealt with systematic forms of oppression around their body or their people being called animals.

These comments were not made in passing on a single occasion but were part of an ongoing pattern of discussion. This graduate student went so far as to document the instances but was hesitant to file a complaint for fear of being labeled a troublemaker and experiencing negative repercussions on her academic career. However, the "smart monkey" comments were made in a disparaging way toward Black students, and the student noted that it was most likely that the white professor making the comments realized how offensive they were in the historical context of the dehumanization of Blacks.

The second and far more egregious incident of blatant racially disparaging comments were made by a professor who insinuated that Black people are lazy and should go back to Africa to sort out their problems there. In this particular case, the student did complain to the administration, and the complaint was dismissed on the grounds that the student was being too sensitive. The incident ended there, with the student realizing that complaining did not help matters and she should just complete her degree and move on.

David also spoke to this inaction on the part of the university:

> One of my professors refuses to provide me with class notes and accessible class reading materials. I reported my concern to the Accessibility Services office, and they told me that there is nothing they could do about it, and I should try and negotiate my accommodations with my professor.

Another recurring aspect of the racial stigmatization were the numerous instances of microaggressions, which were far more common than the disparaging racial comments. First described in a critical race study from the 1970s, a microaggression is a subtle and generally unconscious form of discrimination that makes reference to the deployment of discriminatory stereotypes and expectations as they are made manifest in daily interactions and practices, often in stark contrast to the consciously held or stated principles and beliefs of the one performing the microaggression (Solórzano et al., 2000, p. 62; see also Pierce, 1970). Another related term in relation to subtle enactments of prejudice is "'aversive racism' referring in part to whites' aversion to being seen as prejudiced, given their conscious adherence to egalitarian principles" (DeAngelis, 2009, p. 42). Microaggressions are often unintentional, unconscious, or innocent in their presentation, but in context, the hurtful effects are felt by the students in the form of marginalization and reduced expectations. The majority of the students indicated that they were subjected to microaggressions throughout their academic career.

The subtle nature of microaggression requires greater comprehension of the interaction between the aggressor and the target: "The study of microaggressions looks at the impact of these subtle racial expressions from the perspective of the people being victimized, so it adds to our psychological understanding of the whole process of stigmatization and bias" (DeAngelis, 2009, p. 42). Their concerns about stigmatization are present throughout the interviews. The students' responses yield a plethora of cases of this understated form of racist marginalization.

In one typical example of microaggressions in interactions with professors, Kimberly shares an experience regarding a sociology research project for one of her courses:

> For instance, my initial reason for seeking this advice was because this professor was dealing with methods in terms of "how do you go about doing your research." The conversation ended up becoming a question of my purpose and the impossibilities. There were already assumed limitations before I even really got to express my intent. I didn't even get to see the full breadth of what this study could do. It was spoken with the context of "you can't do this." But I didn't get a why. It's hard to prove.

In cases where the students I spoke with were marginalized in classroom discussions, I repeatedly saw the underestimation of their capability to undertake research and comprehend academic subjects by other students and during office visits with their professors. Lorna, for example, shared, "I think I am judged differently in terms of my intellectual acumen given the fact that I am Black," and when in her study group, "Some of my peers I encountered in a study group were literally unfriendly towards me. I have had to overly justify my research and my opinions. ... I knew the problem was not me or my intellect. It was obvious to me because no other students were treated as a 'problem.'" The student's experiencing of being "judged differently" fits Charles Cooley's (1902) conception of the self. He argues:

> In imagination, we perceive in another's mind some thought of our appearance, manners, aims, deeds, character .... A self-idea of this sort seems to have three principal elements: the imagination of our appearance to the other person; the imagination of his judgement of that appearance; and some sort of self-feeling, such as pride or mortification. (p. 185)

Cooley's statement above is perhaps the most important element in his subsequent theorizing of the self as determined by the "judgment" of oneself by others because this judgment implies some measure by which aspects of the social order impact how we see ourselves positively and negatively. The exercise of judgment is an exercise of power. When that power can be exercised in the consciousness of another—in effect, leading a person to feel ashamed or mortified, to judge themselves in accordance with the judgment of others in a social unit—we are dealing with significant social and political power.

Instead of exercising power physically—controlling others by physical force and compelling their bodies—this conception of the self allows us to understand how power can be exercised so that people self-censure and limit their own options in accordance with social judgment. In other words, the "looking-glass self" (Cooley, 1902) establishes the theoretical foundation for the recognition of the self as a key modality of social and political control.

The idea of the self has probably changed very little from the concept of the looking-glass self as posited by Cooley, a U.S. pioneer in the field of sociology, at the turn of the twentieth century. He theorized this "self" as a sort of manifestation of "self-consciousness" in the social world. In Cooley's (1902) words, "We think of the body as 'I' when it comes to have social function or significance, as when we say 'I am looking well today …' We bring it into the social world, for the time being, and for that reason put our self-consciousness into it" (p. 185). While Cooley (1902), tends to approach the self as a social (and political) construct, his reference to what might be termed the bio-social genesis of the self—the role of our physical bodies, their attributes, and features—should not be overlooked.

As with many microaggressions, these cases are all contextual and it is difficult to establish the offense because often there is no explicit or overt intent to discriminate—it is "micro." In the classroom, again, microaggressions are often subtle, as Denise detailed: "I always notice that when I put my hands up in class they'd go over [not acknowledge] me. And if I have something to say you will cut me off." This theme is repeated in several other interviews.

The University of Toronto is known to the Black disabled students that participated in this research as an institution that publicly celebrates and appreciates its diversity. However, Folake delineates all the elements that set the backdrop for microaggression when she said, "The university likes to brag about how diverse they are, but anti-Black racism is so normalized here such as in the classrooms, with my peers and administration personnel."

At the micro level, the aggressions the Black disabled student experiences can be confounding and confusing. The microaggression contributes to the Black disabled students' disengagement and can motivate them to develop a different perspective on their university experience. The microaggression works by reinforcing what the student perceives as a stigmatization or prejudice inside and outside the classroom. The Black disabled student is made to feel that the classroom is not open to them, and in response, the student may become reclusive from the classroom.

Part of the challenge of addressing racism in an educational institution is that racism has become covert. As overt racism and racial discrimination have become "unfashionable," racism has been forced to assume new forms. As one critic notes, these new forms of anti-Black racism lack the overt signifiers of the past (e.g., racial epithets) but nonetheless subtly continue to define racism in terms of exclusion:

> Apart from the way that racial meanings are inferred rather than stated openly, these new forms are distinguished by the ... closeness it suggests between the idea of race and the ideas of nation, nationalism, and national belonging. We increasingly face a racism which avoids being recognized as such because it is able to link "race" with nationhood, patriotism, and nationalism. (Gilroy, 1999, p. 245)

Gilroy's view of anti-Black racism is not limited to the Canadian context. Indeed, it may be argued that the United States and nations in Europe share a similar experience of living in a paradox: citizens of a racist society that refuses to acknowledge that it is racist (Feagin & Sikes, 1994, 1999). In this context, we must acknowledge the systemic and subtle manifestations of racism and ableism in our society and not be deceived by the superficial signs of "color-blindness." For example, by understanding racism in the sense of systemic discrimination and exclusion, we can recognize individual cases within the broader pattern.

The university's belief that campus diversity establishes the "egalitarian" ideal believed by those who are aversive to racism is evident in the participant interviews. The students in this research encountered these conditions in their daily lives, whether at the hands of their professors or teaching assistants, Accessibility Services administrators, or their non-Black campus peers. In some cases, the comments from members of these groups were blatantly racist.

For example, Christine heard one of her professors clearly stating: "'Black people are all freeloaders,' and he said basically that we should all go back to Africa and work out our problems." Speaking to her reluctance to act against a tenured professor, Christine recounted the advice by the registrar: "I am always told to just suck it up and move on. Suck it up just to get your degree. And the registrar seems to discount the way it was making me feel. You know. I was being abused and nobody cares." The racism went unreported and no action was taken—but the hurtful residual effects remained.

In nearly all of the cases of microaggression, the students indicated a reticence to report because they wanted to avoid trouble or negative consequences for their university standing. As Sarah noted concerning the outrageous "smart monkey" comments:

> I did document the conversations, but I didn't follow through with it because you are so beaten at the end of it all, you don't even have the energy to take people down. You just get to the point where you say, "I am done. Just give me my degree and let me leave."

The failure of the university to take action against microaggressions is excused by claiming oversensitivity on the part of the aggrieved student, as noted by Folake: "I was once called a 'ghetto gal from the poor neighborhood' by another student. I reported the incident to my college registrar, and they told me that I was overreacting." Regardless of the complaint filed by the student to the registrar's office, no one seemed to care about this problem. This is a classic example of the success of colonialism of the mind in which injustice is tacitly accepted by all parties concerned. The microaggression is experienced by the student who, in turn, interprets it to mean that they are not welcome in the classroom, and rather than experiencing personal development and transformation in university, they experience another act of marginalization.

The cumulative effect of these many microaggressions on the study participants was a general sense that the environment at the university was unwelcoming for Black students. Judging from the anecdotal evidence presented during the interviews, there were many more instances than those related, and these incidents had become so commonplace that they were accepted as the reality of university life. Again, students that complained were told they were being too sensitive and that they should tolerate these incidents, obtain their degree, and move on. Only one of the students took a militant attitude and joined a social activist movement.

The insidious nature of microaggression, the subtle contextual signaling and the lack of sufficient proof for action by university authorities or administration left these students with little course of action for relief or validation of their concerns. David ended with a sad commentary on his university experience: "I will leave the university with one thing in my mind: that we'll never be equal, because we're not truly welcome."

The majority of students felt they were treated with contempt and that the near universal opinion of the professors was that the academic accommodations provided an undue advantage to the Black disabled students, and that their success was largely due to the facilitation of these accommodations. Again, the descriptor of stigmatization was applied to their experience. Many of the students were reluctant to enroll with Accessibility Services for fear of this stigmatization. Thus, the students felt marginalized by their treatment as Black disabled students due to anti-Black racism and contempt for the accommodations afforded disabled students.

Stigmatization is quite powerful, and it can have implications for the personal growth and development of the stigmatized. In the higher education setting, the experience of stigmatization will contribute to marginalization through the assumptions, attitudes, and both micro and macro social relations of the Black disabled students. Subsequently, marginalization of the student is produced through the student's experience in the classroom and with administrators. The intersectional nature of marginalization is such that it can have implications for the identity of the student and lead to a negative impact for the personal growth of the student.

Sometimes, the students either chose to ignore the racism or to embrace their ethnicity and surround it with pride. Saga used the perceived disadvantage of being Black to his advantage and to confront racism head-on, educating himself by being an avid reader and then joining an organization that actively fights anti-Black racism:

> I found other people at the university who have struggled in similar ways like me. I've always found myself, like, people would say that "he's smart." Or I think I'm smart because I'm inclined to like reading a lot. I am more comfortable in carrying on an intellectual conversation. I have a thirst for gaining knowledge. I've been treated differently even by my own people [Black people] at the university. Having the experience of being around Black students on campus, I feel honored to be in that circle. Many people consider me strange; my own Black people. I might be seen as a strange person. I can be a bit critical about certain things. I am definitely seen as a shit disturber because I am also a member of a social movement.

Saga's statement is particularly interesting because we see here how a Black disabled student draws close connections between the struggles against ableism and anti-Black racism. I believe Saga's statement is particularly significant because it is an experience that one encounters again and again: people with disabilities feel a particular affinity to the struggle against stigma or discrimination. As a Black person, I believe this sense of affinity is connected to the way the bodies of individuals with disabilities are subject to discipline and definition by medical and educational institutions and the government. There are analogous to way the bodies of Black people were enslaved and controlled. In taking pride in his intellect and being a "shit disturber," Saga's terms can be understood as behaviors of self-care.

The shape that Blackness should take is also a matter of discussion among researchers. Lynn (2004) outlined the debate among scholarly researchers about the extent to which race should be accepted as a critical pedagogy and how it is that Blackness fits into schooling and society. She notes that, there has been substantial growth in how schooling and society are viewed in the scope of academic study and that, through the application of critical investigation, it is possible to develop a stronger understanding of how Blackness is nested in social research. Schooling is an area of specific interest because of the necessity to understand the approach schooling and education has taken toward Black students. Through the current scholarly research on Black identity, it is possible to develop a stronger understanding of the impacts of administration on the role Blackness plays in the accommodations that students expect and experience at the university level.

Black identity, in such formulations, is always a site of contestation because of the awareness of one's double consciousness, or when considering sexuality, a thirdness. This remains an important mode of critically thinking about the subject here, and it shapes what I am calling the "more classic" notion of identity-based resistance. This fits with the overall theme of marginality. That is because, through the double consciousness described by DuBois, Black people experience marginalization due to identity.

The challenge for society goes beyond dismantling a system that supports ableism and anti-Black racism to the point that the vestiges of these phenomenon could be removed. It also requires a fundamental change to how people view the Black person. We are seen as a problem though we ask for little compared to what we can offer society. Black people are capable of doing great things; however, the current structure of our institutions prevent us from achieving our potential. Black people are stuck behind in a system that does not support their performance or growth as people. The systems are adapted to white middle-class able-bodied students, and they do not respond well to the problems and barriers faced by Black disabled students. For instance, my experience was one where both microaggressions within the policy and procedure of the school as well as similar but not always unconscious racist and ableist attitudes of faculty and administration threatened my ability to succeed as a student.

As Levchak (2018) notes, racial microaggressions are symptomatic of the broader social problem of white supremacist thought, institutional anti-Black racism, and hatred that fuels racially motivated macroaggressions, bullying, intimidation, harassment, and violence. Systemic oppression by white supremacy was evident at every turn in my attempts at academic advancement and success. All too often it contributed to the violence and racial trauma of being a Black man in academia. The paternalistic and plantation mentality of the university and its agents were disruptive to my experience and, as my primary research indicates, they have been disruptive for several other students at the institution as well (McKittrick, 2013; Walcott, 2021). Current and past scholarly work, as well as the narratives of Black people over the past two centuries, all present a consistent theme of those in power seeking to maintain that power by imposing a hierarchy, offering social assistance with strings attached and help from agents of a white supremacist system.

Many North American institutions, including the education system, are steeped in anti-Blackness and anti-Black racism. Colonized educational institutions preserve and perpetuate a system of structured inequality based on Blackness, disability, gender (Collins, 2015; Dei, 2022; McKittrick, 2015; Pickens, 2019; Wynter, 2003), placing special value on non-racialized, able-bodied, males. Thus, the university system carries vestiges of what education was designed to accomplish: preparing privileged people for success and marginalized people for disappointment. Barriers persist for Black disabled students who must struggle to overcome to obtain a place in an education program and to be successful in these programs. At both secondary and postsecondary levels, there is considerable institutional resistance to full inclusion and equitably accessible education for Black students or students with disabilities. This education is, of course, critical not only to personal and intellectual growth and development but also to attaining economic self-sufficiency.

As Fanon (1967) notes, racism and colonialism depend in no small way on Euro-American power convincing Black people of their own inferiority. In many such cases, even the Black man believes that white is the color of power and acceptance (p. 9). White being the "default" renders people of other races, cultures, and heritages inherently flawed or diminished. In a very subtle yet important way, we can see that the power of the university lies in its capacity to not only project and support power but also to conceal it.

Surveillance

The students I spoke with felt discriminated against, and while each had their own unique lived experiences, as people who are both Black and disabled, they shared the experience of cross-sectional marginalization, with the system and its agents acting in ways that were both racist and ableist. My own lived experience was similar. My department chair's antagonistic behavior was distressing. Though my only objective was intellectual growth, I was left to feel as though I was a complex problem that needed to be solved. Her behavior toward me was not consistent with her behavior toward white students. The system supported her behavior; she was able to have security monitor and surveil my activities, even though there was no reason to believe I was taking advantage of my access to assistive technology in the building for anything other than work. Anti-Black racism was implicit in the way the university treated me and the Black students who were interviewed.

Anti-Blackness or anti-Black racism and fear of Black men are not exclusive to white individuals. Anti-Blackness is not just about the racial oppression, prejudice, and discrimination against Black people by white people; it comes from other racial and ethnic groups as well, all of whom have themselves been heavily influenced by white supremacist ideologies (Comrie et al., 2022, p. 75). I share Fanon's (1967) and Ibram X Kendi's (2020) view that a person is either racist or antiracist, and there is nothing in between. It is noteworthily exhausting to ask how one inhuman behavior can differ from another inhuman behavior. All forms of anti-Blackness resemble one another. The person who is dehumanized is dehumanized, and it is an awful thing to experience.

It is dangerous to ascribe to this sense of Blackness, which is created by the European oppressor, the Blackness that is dehumanized. The systemic nature of anti-Blackness is important, especially for people in positions of authority and especially where one's freedom depends on being treated with justice and equity. Browne (2015) argues that surveillance is the lived experiences of Blackness in "which surveillance is practiced, narrated," and normalized through acts of violence (p. 9). She also points out that it is "the organizational framework of our present human condition that names what is and what is not bounded within the category of the human, and that fixes and frames Blackness as an object of surveillance" (p. 8). The system was inhabited by staff in such a way that their anti-Black racism and ableist attitudes were rationalized. Researchers have found that Black student experiences reveal a normalization of anti-Blackness on Canadian university campuses—microaggressions, prejudice, harassment, policing, violent threats, and even blatant disregard by some professors—most of which are often dismissed by those in positions of power and the university as a whole (Cameron & Jefferies, 2021, pp. 4–5; see also Bell et al., 2020).

That I am a Black man is not an acceptable rationale for the behavior of staff who treated me as though I do not belong in spaces of higher education. My completion of degree programs at the baccalaureate and master's levels is evidence that I am a scholar engaged in learning. Accomplishing this level of education should have been evidence enough of my ability, and I should not have to worry about staff or security monitoring and surveilling my activities. Without evidence that I could pose a threat to the safety and security of the institution, it is simply anti-Black racism and an assumption that, because of *the skin I am in*, I do not belong in the university environment.

Fiske (1998) argues that surveillance is a way of enforcing normalcy "where those who have been marginalized in to the 'abnormal' have surveillance focused more intensely upon them" (p. 81). This statement is exemplified by my encounter with the department chair, where surveillance reinforced my inferior status of Blackness and disability in the university (Browne, 2015; Lyon et al., 2012).

My accomplishments and documented progress on my doctoral project should stand as reason enough to accept that I was completing my project in earnest; however, given the design of the education system and the attitudes of staff, I was subject to marginalization on par with someone who had done nothing to earn the trust of the system and its agents. I am not the only one, however. My experiences and those of the students I interviewed should be reflected upon as further evidence of how racist biases permeate the university's administrative structure and are made flesh through the behavior of faculty, administration, and security staff. This is a disappointing finding, but like other findings in my research, it appears to be common in academic institutions.

Given my research findings, one may legitimately question whether the institution really wants Black students to enroll in their universities. Canadian university discourse on inclusion does pay lip service to the ideas of equity and mutual respect for Black students. However, the discourse of inclusion is a form of concealment that obscures the underlying structural marginalization of significant portions of the university population. The marginalization of Black students in universities can be seen as a form of cultural racism that may be defined as a network of beliefs and attitudes that justify discriminatory practices. A common example of this cultural racism is the representation of the "problem" of Black students.

It is difficult to speculate based on these findings alone, or even in light of other peripheral research in the area of anti-Black racism and ableism in educational institutions, why the system continues to work as it does, even while academics and professionals are cognizant that these problems exist and that there must be a concerted response to them for there to be a satisfactory conclusion to this problem. As Mitchell and Snyder (2000) noted, "Nearly every culture views disability as a problem in need of a solution" (p. 47); which I would extend to Blackness as well.

Previous literature and the findings of the current research suggest that this is a consistent sentiment for the academy. The education system is designed in such a way that policy and procedure are structured as though Blackness and disabled people are problems that must be solved. While there is a belief that effort must be taken to accommodate me and to support my plea for accommodation, there must be documentation and bureaucracy that confirms that I require assistance. The agent of the system too often perpetuates the stigma of the disabled student, even when the student requires only simple accommodations to ensure equal access with able-bodied students.

This research reveals Black disabled students perception that faculty will often marginalize them and their requirements. This is a violation of the principle of educational justice, which states that engaged students willing to learn should have reasonable accommodations. As a Black man, I am *not* a problem in *need* of a solution, I am a student in *need* of accommodation because I am made to function in a system that does not imagine Blackness and disability as essential to its way of being.

While students with disabilities struggle for inclusion and reasonable accommodations, another struggle is occurring sub-textually: the struggle to define their identity and to learn who they are as people with disabilities. As a Black man, I am particularly cognizant of issues of discrimination and prejudice, and for this reason, the students' experiences have expanded my understanding of the struggles for access and equity in our society.

While there was no good reason to justify the harassment and surveilling I experienced, there is also evidence that other Black students have had similar experiences. There have been recent instances of anti-Black racism and harassment in higher education institutions in both Canada and United States.

For example, in June 2019, a Black student with a 9.0 GPA at the University of Ottawa was subjected to anti-Black racism by security guards because he was without his student identification card at the time. The student said he was skateboarding when the guards stopped him and asked for his ID. He told the guards he didn't have his wallet on him, and he tried to walk away, but the guards followed him and knocked his phone to the ground, which he was using to record the incident. As a result, the student was grabbed, carded, arrested for trespassing on private property, and forced to sit handcuffed on a campus street for two hours (Ramlakhan, 2019).

Similarly, Jordan, a law student at the University of Windsor, says he was confronted with what it means to be a Black student on a campus in Canada, and the reality of what that means scares him. On February 14, 2019, Jordon, a Black male student, was running late for a class at the Odette Building on the university campus. When he opened the door, he hit another student, who was white or white-passing (Tomlinson et al., 2021). When this student pushed Jordon, Jordon punched the other student back. This event was investigated by the university and, while both students complained under the University of Windsor Student Non-Academic Misconduct Policy, Jordon was banned from campus days after meeting with the Academic Integrity and Student Conduct Officer and the other student was free to use the campus as he wished (Tomlinson et al., 2021). He adds that he began to see in real-time what anti-Black racism can do to our lives. It can mean the difference between being a lawyer and being a criminal (Tomlinson et al., 2021).

Similarly, a white Yale University student saw a Black graduate student sleeping in the common room of their dorm and called the police, effectively racially profiling her. The student was interrogated by campus police officers and carded (Griggs, 2018, p. 1). In another incident, Black students from the University of Florida celebrating their graduation were violently grabbed and pushed offstage by a U.S. Marshal (Wootson, 2018).

In each of these cases, Black students were treated as though they do not belong in spaces of higher education. These incidents suggest that institutions of higher education have a pattern of practicing and/or facilitating anti-Black racism, serving to highlight the symbolic status of Blackness as a form of outsiderness (Bhabha, 1994; Durham, 2020; Mignolo, 2012).

Anti-Black racism is ingrained in the hearts and minds of some people, and having economic, political, and class privilege over certain people is a potent recipe for reinforcing racism and exclusion in higher education. Walcott (2021) notes that the death of George Floyd, an unarmed Black man in the United States, "affirmed what many Black people like me already knew: that we have a different relationship to property [such as in higher education institutions] and its meaning than white people and many other people of color do" (p. 12). This should not come as a surprise to anyone. He also writes that because Floyd's death was caught on camera, it helped reveal how Black people are constantly targeted and surveilled by self-appointed white authorities. "These recordings of Black bodies have become a genre of their own, whereby 'Karen' or 'Amy' refuse to let Black people live their lives, with all the assumptions about Blackness and property integral to these interactions" (p. 30).

The cornerstone of these self-appointed white authorities is the act of white supremacy, which is rooted in anti-Black racism in subtle and complex ways. As Levchak (2018) reminds us, anti-Black racism is embedded in the everyday experiences of Black students "when they are watched, followed, or surveilled by members of the academic community and law enforcement as though [we] are dangerous or don't belong" (p. 26).

In particular, these injuries are, of course, the product of a general practice of anti-Black racist culture that normalizes the violence, surveillance, assaults, and isolation of Black students in these institutions (Browne, 2015; Fanon, 1967; McKittrick, 2011; Walcott, 2021). However, given the violence worked on Black male bodies in society, there is irony in the fact that Black people looking to the university to acquire the tools to do better in the world face the same dangers in the academy. Cole (2020) notes that "institutions in today's white supremacist settler colonial context always come in peace and goodwill. They always tell us they mean well, and thus they refuse to own their endless violence against Black people" (p. 7).

Walcott (2016) holds that "Black life is lived in the constant … [danger] of violence on the road to death" (p. 192), highlighting the many lives of Black men who end up murdered. Fanon (1963) argues that "violence … governed the order of the colonial world" and that the initial contact between oppressor and oppressed was "colored by violence" (p. 50), concluding that it is only logical that violence is necessary to conclude this process. For Fanon, this is the counterviolence of anticolonial struggles. Collins (2017) observes, "Social institutions routinely [reproduce] power hierarchies where violence is vested less in speech but rather in bureaucratic action and custom" (p. 1463). I would argue that institutions are, by definition, sociopolitical constructions created and maintained by violence to ensure the power structure and control—including control over Black lives.

Ultimately, this stigmatizing process explains, at least in part, the deep cultural fear of Black men that informs Western culture to this very day. Fanon wrote over 60 years ago about the treatment of Black men as threatening simply by reason of theirs Blackness and thus sinfulness. He recounts traveling on a train in Paris in the 1950s when he painfully experienced the physical reality of his colonized body "as one that has always already been transformed by the negative stereotypes placed upon [his Blackness], into a subhuman reality" (Fanon, 1967, as cited in Wynter, 1999, p. 21; Wynter et al., 2020). When a young white boy sees him and then points at him and cries to his mother, "Mama, see the Negro! I'm frightened!," he realizes, "Now they were beginning to be afraid of me" (Fanon, 1967, p. 112). However, Black individuals today still internalize—to a significant degree—the psychosocial and visible representations of our Blackness as a force that is inherently disruptive and threatening to the social order.

In social space, as Goffman (1967) observes, we all live within a "world of social encounters" (p. 21). In the course of these encounters, an individual—as a social self—attempts to "act out" a particular pattern of behaviors by which those the individual interacts with gain an impression of the individual. He contends that it does not really matter if a person intends to act out these behaviors or not, the end result is the same in that people gain an overall image of the person.

The faculty and administration in North American universities behave in a way that is entirely consistent with one another and Black students should be prepared for a system that requires them to deal with mentors and school administrators who create barriers and pressures that non-racialized people do not face. This is an unacceptable, albeit common, occurrence. We must all work and live our lives in a culture that—for Black people and people with disabilities—defines and regulates our identities. Nonetheless, there is the possibility that we can define spaces in the margins where we can make our own language, culture, and discourse and assume control of who we are as people.

The racist and ableist attitudes of agents of higher education are supported by the policies and procedures entrenched within its bureaucracy, just as the policies and procedures embedded within the bureaucracy of the system support the racist and ableist attitudes of its agents. This is an iterative phenomenon, and even as there are often minimum efforts by those within the system to provide examples of change, the generally held perception that change has happened within the system is just as detrimental to the Black student as the system's structure and agent's attitudes are to the success of students working within it.

Substantial change cannot happen without fundamentally dismantling and realigning the system and the attitudes of its agents. Black people can no longer be perceived as problems that require solutions; they must be appreciated for the diverse lived experiences and abilities they bring to the classroom. The system must be designed to accommodate needs, not to stigmatize those who have needs. Black students should not be treated as potential criminals that require monitoring, and staff should not rely on bureaucracy as a rationale for racist treatment of students. The current paradigm simply does not support the achievement of equality, and the nature of the changes required to get to that point remain quite far from being realized. The cultural norm of people with disabilities being seen as problems in need of solutions "situates people with disabilities in a profoundly ambivalent relation to the cultures and stories they inhabit" (Mitchell & Snyder, 2000, p. 47). Successful change must confront this deeply embedded racist and ableist side of North American culture if successful transformation is to happen.

References

Accessibility for Ontarians with Disabilities Act. (2023). *Accessible supervision of graduate students with disabilities.* https://www.aoda.ca/accessible-supervision-of-graduate-students-with-disabilities/.

Baptist, J., Minnie, L., Buksner, S., Kaye, R., & Morgan, J. (2007). Screening in the early years for mathematics difficulties and disabilities: Identifying red flags to support early learners at risk. *Orbit, 37*(1).

Barnes, M., & Wade-Wooley, L. (2007). Where there's a will there are ways to close the achievement gap for children with learning difficulties. *Orbit, 37*(1).

Becker, H. (1963). *Outsiders: Studies in the sociology of deviance.* Free Press.

Bell, L. A. (2003). Telling tales: What stories can teach us about racism. *Race, Ethnicity and Education, 6*(1), 3–28.

Bell, M. P., Berry, D., Leopold, J., & Nkomo, S. (2020). Making Black lives matter inacademia: A Black feminist call for collective action against anti-blackness in the academy. *Gender, Work and Organization, 28*(S1), 39–57. https://doi.org/10.1111/gwao.12555

Bhabha, H. K. (1994). *The location of culture.* Routledge.

Browne, S. (2015). *Dark matters: On the surveillance of blackness.* Duke University Press.

Butler, J. (1993). *Bodies that matter: On the discursive limits of "sex."* Routledge.

Butler, J., & Athanasiou, A. (2013). *Dispossession: The performative in the political*. John Wiley & Sons.

Cameron, E. S., & Jefferies, K. (2021). Anti-Black racism in Canadian education: A call to action to support the next generation. *Healthy Populations Journal, 1*(1).

Cahill, A. J. (2000). Foucault, rape, and the construction of the feminine body. *Hypatia, 15*(1), 43–63.

Cole, D. (2020). *The skin we're in*. Doubleday Canada.

Collins, P. H. (1990). *Black feminist thought: Knowledge, consciousness, and the politics of empowerment*. Unwin Hyman.

Collins, P. H. (2015). Intersectionality's definitional dilemmas. *Annual Review of Sociology*. 41, 1–20.

Collins, P. H. (2017). On violence, intersectionality and transversal politics. *Ethnic and Racial Studies, 40*(9), 1460–1473.

Comrie, J. W., Landor, A. M., Riley, K. T., & Williamson, J. D. (2022). Anti-Blackness/Colorism. In *Moving toward antibigotry*. Boston University, Center for Antiracism Research. https://www.bu.edu/antiracism-center/files/2022/06/Anti-Black.pdf.

Connor, D., Ferri, B. & Annamma, S. (2016). *Discrit: Disability studies and critical race theory in education*. Teachers College Press.

Conrad, P. (1975). The discovery of hyperkinesis: Notes on the medicalization of deviant behaviour. *Social Problems, 23*(1), 12–21.

Cooley, C. (1902). *Human nature and the social order*. Charles Scribner's Sons.

Davis, L. J. (1995). *Enforcing normalcy: Disability, deafness, and the body*. Verso Books.

DeAngelis, T. (2009). Unmaskin' racial microaggressions. *Monitor on Psychology, 40*(2), 42.

Dei, G. J. S. (2022). Cosmopolitanism or multiculturalism? Towards an anti-colonial reading. *International Journal for Talent Development and Creativity, 10*(1), 31–44.

Dolmage, J. (2017). *Academic ableism: Disability and higher education*. University of Michigan Press.

Douglas, P., & Martino, A. S. (2020). Introduction: Disability studies in education—Critical conversations. *Canadian Journal of Disability Studies, 9*(5), 1–19.

Du Bois, W. E. B. (1903). *The souls of black folk*. A.C. McClurg & Co.

Durham, A. (2020). Black feminist thought, intersectionality, and intercultural communication. *Intersectionality: Race, intercultural communication, and politics*, 45–57.

Fanon, F. (1961). The pitfalls of national consciousness by. In *The Wretched of the Earth*. Grove Press. Retrieved from: https://www.marxists.org/subject/africa/fanon/pitfalls-national.htm.

Fanon, F. (1963). *The wretched of the earth*. Grove Press.

Fanon, F. (1967). *Black skin, white masks*. Trans. Charles Lam Markmann. Grove Press.

Feagin, J. R., & Sikes, M. P. (1994). *Living with racism: The black middle-class experience*. Beacon Press.

Feagin, J. R. & Sikes, M. P. (1999). Changing the colour line: The future of U.S. racism. In Martin Bulmer & John Solomos (Eds.), *Racism* (pp. 407–411). Oxford University Press.

Ferri, B. A., & Connor, D. J. (2006). Challenging normalcy: Dis/ability, race, and the normalized classroom. In *Reading resistance: Discourses of exclusion in desegregation and inclusion* debates (pp. 127–143). Peter Lang.

Finkelstein, V. (2007). *The social model of disability and the disability movement.* https://disability-studies.leeds.ac.uk/wp-content/uploads/sites/40/library/finkelstein-The-Social-Model-of-Disability-and-the-Disability-Movement.pdf.

Fiske, J. (1998). Surveilling the city: Whiteness, the black man and democratic totalitarianism. *Theory, Culture & Society, 15*(2), 67–88.

Fleming, V. (Director). (1939). *The Wizard of Oz* [Film]. Metro-Goldwyn-Mayer.

Foster, J. (2007). Cultivating gifted students: How parents and teachers can support exceptional learners. *Orbit, 37*(1), 36–40.

Foucault, M. (1978). *The history of sexuality: Volume I.* Trans. R. Hurley. Pantheon Books.

Foucault, M. (1995). *Discipline and punish: The birth of the prison.* Trans. Alan Sheridan. Random House.

Garland-Thomson, R. (1997). *Extraordinary bodies: Figuring physical disability in American culture and literature.* Columbia University Press.

Gates, H. L., Jr. (1986). Race as the trope of the world. In *Race, writing and difference* (pp. 1–20). University of Chicago Press.

Gilroy, P. (1999). The end of anti-racism. In M. Bulmer & J. Solomos (Eds.), *Racism* (pp. 242–250). Oxford University Press.

Gilroy, P. (2000). *Between camps: Race, identity, and nationalism at the end of the colour line.* Penguin Press.

Gilroy, P. (2005). *Postcolonial melancholia.* Columbia University Press.

Goffman, E. (1967). *Interaction ritual: Essays on face-to-face behavior.* Anchor Books.

Goodley, D. (2014). *Dis/ability studies: Theorising disablism and ableism.* Routledge.

Goodley, D., Lawthom, R., Liddiard, K., & Runswick-Cole, K. (2019). Provocations for critical disability studies. *Disability & Society, 34*(6), 972–997.

Griggs, B. (2018, May 12). A black Yale graduate student took a nap in her dorm's common room. So a white student called police. *CNN.com.* Retrieved from https://www.cnn.com/2018/05/09/us/yale-student-napping-black-trnd/index.html.

Hall, S. (2001). Negotiating Caribbean identities. In B. Meeks & F. Lindahl (Eds.), *New Caribbean thought: A reader* (pp. 24–39). University of the West Indies Press.

Hanisch, C. (2006). *The personal is political: The women's liberation movement classic with a new explanatory introduction.* http://webhome.cs.uvic.ca/~mserra/AttachedFiles/PersonalPolitical.pdf.

Hegel, G. (2019). *Georg Wilhelm Friedrich Hegel: The phenomenology of spirit.* Cambridge, New York, Port Melbourne, New Delhi, Singapore: Cambridge University Press.

hooks, b. (1992). *Black looks: Race and representation.* South End Press.

Kannen, V. (2008). Identity treason: Race, disability, queerness, and the ethics of (post) identity practices. *Culture, Theory and Critique, 49*(2), 149–163.

Kendi, I. X. (2020). Ibram X Kendi defines what it means to be an antiracist. *Penguin.co.uk.* Retrieved from https://www.penguin.co.uk/articles/2020/06/ibram-x-kendi-definition-of-antiracist.

Kgatla, S. (2018). The decolonisation of the mind. Black consciousness community projects by the Limpopo Council of Churches. *Missionalia, 46*, 146–162. Available at: https://doi.org/10.7832/46-1-270.

Kuusisto, S. (2018). *Planet of the blind. It's not as dark as you think*: Structural inequality at Syracuse University. https://stephenkuusisto.com/2018/04/29/7735/

Levchak, C. C. (2018). Microaggressions, macroaggressions, and modern racism in higher education. In *Microaggressions and modern racism* (pp. 85–104). Palgrave Macmillan.

Linton, S. (1998). *Claiming disability: Knowledge and identity*. New York University Press.

Lorde, A. (1984). *Sister outsider: Essays and speeches*. Crossing Press.

Lynn, M. (2004). Inserting the race into critical pedagogy: An analysis of race-based epistemologies. *Educational Philosophy and Theory, 36*(2), 153–165.

Lyon, D., Ball, K., & Haggerty, K. D. (Eds.). (2012). *Routledge handbook of surveillance studies*. Routledge.

McKittrick, K. (2000). Who do you talk to, when a body's in trouble? M. Nourbese Philip's (un)silencing of black bodies in the diaspora. *Social & Cultural Geography, 1*(2), 223–236.

McKittrick, K. (2011). On plantations, prisons, and a black sense of place. *Social & Cultural Geography, 12*(8), 947–963.

McKittrick, K. (2013). Plantation futures. *Small Axe, 17*(3), 1–15.

McKittrick, K. (Ed.). (2015). *Sylvia Wynter: On being human as praxis*. Duke University Press.

McKittrick, K. (2016). Diachronic loops/deadweight tonnage/bad made measure. *Cultural Geographies, 23*(1), 3–18.

Johnson, M. L., & McRuer, R. (2024). Cripistemologies now (more than ever!). *Journal of Literary & Cultural Disability Studies, 18*(2), 115–134.

Michalko, R. (2002). *The difference that disability makes*. Temple University Press.

Mignolo, W. D. (2012). *Local histories/global designs: Coloniality, subaltern knowledges, and border thinking*. Princeton University Press.

Mitchell, D. T., & Snyder, S. L. (2000). *Narrative prosthesis: Disability and the dependencies of discourse*. University of Michigan Press.

Morgan, J. (2023). On the relationship between race and disability. *The Harvard Civil Rights-Civil Liberties Law Review, 58*, 663. Retrieved from https://journals.law.harvard.edu/crcl/wp-content/uploads/sites/80/2023/09/HLC202_Morgan.pdf.

Muñoz, J. E. (1999). *Disidentifications: Queers of color and the performance of politics*. University of Minnesota Press.

Oliver, M. (1996). *Understanding disability: From theory to practice*. St. Martin's Press.

Oelofsen, R. (2015). Decolonisation of the African mind and intellectual landscape. *Phronimon, 1616*(2), 130–146.

Pickens, T. A. (2019). *Black madness:: Mad blackness*. Duke University Press.

Pierce, C. (1970). Offensive mechanisms: The vehicle for microaggressions. In F. Barbour (Ed.), *The Black seventies* (pp. 265–282). Porter Sargent.

Ramlakhan, K. (2019, June 14). Black student carded, cuffed at University of Ottawa, prompting review. *CBC News.* https://www.cbc.ca/news/canada/ottawa/university-human-rights-office-student-twitter-carding-1.5175864.

Sandahl, C. (2004). Black man, blind man: Disability, identity, politics and performance. *Theatre Journal, 56*(4), 579–602.

Shakespeare, T., & Watson, N. (2002). The social model of disability: An outdated ideology? In *Exploring theories and expanding methodologies: Where we are and where we need to go* (pp. 9–28). Emerald Group Publishing.

Solórzano, D., Ceja, M., & Yosso, T. (2000). Critical race theory, racial microaggressions, and campus racial climate: The experiences of African American college students. *Journal of Negro Education, 69*(1–2), 60–73.

Taylor, S. (2011). Beasts of burden: Disability studies and animal rights. *Qui Parle: Critical Humanities and Social Sciences, 19*(2), 191–222.

Thomas-Long, R. (2010). *The politics of exclusion in graduate education.* Peter Lang.

Titchkosky, T. (2000). Disability studies: The old and the new. *Canadian Journal of Sociology, 25*(2), 197–224.

Titchkosky, T. (2003). *Disability, self, and society.* University of Toronto Press.

Titchkosky, T. (2007). *Reading and writing disability differently: The textured life of embodiment.* University of Toronto Press.

Titchkosky, T. (2011). *The question of access: Disability, space, meaning.* University of Toronto Press.

Titchkosky, T. (2015). Life with dead metaphors: Impairment rhetoric in social justice praxis. *Journal of Literary & Cultural Disability Studies, 9*(1), 1–18.

Titchkosky, T., & Michalko, R. (2009). *Rethinking normalcy: A disability studies reader.* Canadian Scholars' Press.

Tomlinson, A., Mayor, L., & Baksh, N. (2021, February 24). Being Black on campus: Why students, staff and faculty say universities are failing them. *CBC News.* https://www.cbc.ca/news/canada/anti-black-racism-campus-university-1.5924548

Walcott, R. (2003). *Black like who? Writing Black Canada.* Insomniac Press.

Walcott, R. (2016). *Queer returns: Essays on multiculturalism, diaspora, and black studies.* Insomniac Press.

Walcott, R. (2021). *On property: Policing, prisons, and the call for abolition* (Vol. 2). Biblioasis.

Weber, M., Henderson, A. M., & Parsons, T. (1947). *The theory of social and economic organization.* Oxford University Press.

Wootson, C. R., Jr. (2018, May 7). Black students celebrating their graduation say a marshal shoved them away from the stage. *Washington Post.* Retrieved from https://www.washingtonpost.com/news/grade-point/wp/2018/05/07/black-students-celebrating-their-graduation-say-a-marshal-shoved-them-away-from-the-stage/?utm_term=.7c5bf9484cea.

Wotherspoon, T. (2014). *The sociology of education in Canada: Critical perspectives* (4th ed.). Oxford University Press.

Wynter, S. (1994, Fall). No humans involved: An open letter to my colleagues. In *Forum N.H.I.: Knowledge for the 21st Century: Knowledge on Trial, 1*(1), 42–73.

Wynter, S. (1999). *Towards the sociogenic principle: Fanon, the puzzle of conscious experience, of identity and what it's like to be black*. http://coribe.org/PDF/wynter_socio.pdf.

Wynter, S. (2003). Unsettling the coloniality of being/power/truth/freedom: Towards the human, after man, its overrepresentation—An argument. *CR: The New Centennial Review, 3*(3), 257–337.

Wynter, S., Bennett, J., & Givens, J. R. (2020). "A greater truth than any other truth you know": A conversation with professor Sylvia Wynter on Origin Stories. *Souls (Boulder, Colo.), 22*(1), 123–137. Retrieved from https://doi.org/10.1080/10999949.2020.1811592.

Chapter 5

Accommodations

To arrange accommodations, all of the students interviewed sought services through the Accessibility Services office. At times, the desire to avoid the stigmatization associated with societal views on disability, and with the use of academic accommodations, conflicted directly with their educational needs for these services. Several of the students delayed accessing these services, trying to get by without the accommodations.

This conflict between the need to fit into society and avoid stigma and the educational need for accommodations speaks to the discrimination Black disabled students experience at the University of Toronto by staff and professor who are prejudiced against disabled students. This experience of stigma made many of the participants trepidatious regarding signing up for accommodations through the Accessibility Services office.

It is crucial to understand the power aspect of the accommodations; for some students, the accommodations are vital to their ability to achieve in their classrooms. The power the institution holds to withhold or delay the disbursement of the accommodations can adversely affect the students' performance in the classroom. As noted by Folake, whose accommodations were delayed:

> I had great difficulties accessing accommodations, such as getting a voice recorder, laptop, and assistive technology to help with my studies. When I applied to Accessibility Services Office for bursaries to buy assistive technology, it takes them months (four months or more) to approve the bursary. Sometimes, when I received the bursary, the seminar is already finished which means I may have to give the money back.

She noted that the power the institution has over disabled students is great in and of itself, and withholding the necessary accommodations can create its own set of problems in confronting the power structure. In severe cases, the experience can be much more than an annoyance; it can mean the end of an academic endeavor.

Barry did not conform to the system, and it cost him, "I was left in the dark and as a result ... dropped out of school for one academic year." The system of assessing students to determine academic accommodation needs was not always a negative experience; however, the students did encounter shortcomings and inherent biases that were a source of frustration, as can be expected when dealing with the bureaucracy of the university. David, reflecting upon his experiences with Accessibility Services, notes:

> I have had a great experience thus far accessing accommodations with the Accessibility Services office. The only issue I had is the design of the learning assessment tests. I believe the process of the learning assessment test is culturally framed. I also believe that the learning assessment tests are too long, and they're designed so that each student fails. It doesn't a give fair or accurate reflection of the person's actual ability. I have low vision, which I informed the psychoeducational assessment administrator of before the assessment, but still all of the testing materials were in small prints. The learning assessment administrator only gave me five or ten minutes to complete a task.

Max Weber (1947) once argued that the depersonalization of work processes successfully eliminates personal feelings from decision-making in bureaucratic organizations. This means that, rationally, decisions made in a bureaucracy will be based on what will maintain the system; the bureaucracy depersonalizes itself from humanistic considerations. Because bureaucratic policies permeate most modern institutions, these policies have become normal elements of the way institutions work. Bureaucracy becomes a social problem to the extent to which it supports marginalization and discrimination.

The self-identification required for the Accessibility Services application does not capture the complexity of the identity process. For instance, learning assessment forms and Accessibility Services forms for both the undergraduate and graduate levels make identity issues increasingly problematic for Black students with disabilities, as noted in previous chapters by the participants. This "identity" is crafted from both the students' self-description of their introspective racial self-assessment and the disability identity that is assigned to them by the university or medical professionals. The issue of how disability should actually be addressed by administrators is a difficult one because of how disability is conceptualized. Titchkosky (2011) recognizes that the nature of how disability is handled at the level of organizational bureaucracy is such that the classification of disability includes the inabilities of disabled students and restrictions from activities. Practices at the university level recognize disability as an aspect related to the framing of time and the way daily life is structured. Titchkosky does this through analysis of the history of ordinary narratives that reflect on the perpetuation of presence and absence of disability exclusion and inclusion. She describes how disability is an issue for inclusion, and she concludes this based on the idea of disability as a present factor, which bureaucracies address as though the issue is not-yet present. Titchkosky's work presents further evidence of the way bureaucracies address the conditions in which disability is considered and the way bureaucracy is addressed in the classroom from the standpoint of the way considerations of bureaucracies are perpetuated in the education system. For example, for a disabled student, the stigma of disability contributes to the design of policies in a school that values standardized tests, which may have discriminatory elements embedded in them. As they are necessary parts of decision-making, this could impact placement and acceptance for students. The accommodations are dependent upon the assessment tests administered by Accessibility Services, a capitulation to the power held by the institution requiring that they surrender their individuality to the commonality of a uniform discipline and label marking them with symbolic submission. Thus, society has continued to be bureaucratic and to develop ways to detach emotion from decision-making and create further bureaucratization in the systems and processes of institutional environments (Weber, 1947). The structure of bureaucracy creates difficulties for disabled and Black individuals as university students. These difficulties are related to the future university bureaucracy adequately developing policy to meet particular students' needs. This embeds discrimination into the system that could address their personal needs. The difficulties for these students are related to their needs for specific adjustments that the bureaucracy, as an impersonal and "rational" system, did not recognize or acknowledge.

Plantation Mentality in Accessibility

The University of Toronto has an expressed policy of commitment to provide accessibility for all students, regardless of disability. According to its statement on the Accessibility Services website:

> The University will strive to provide support for and facilitate the accommodation of individuals with disabilities so that all may share the same level of access to opportunities, participate in the full range of activities that the University offers, and achieve their full potential as members of the University community. (UofT, 2023, p. 1)

This affirmation for all students is a lofty goal, but it does not appear to be manifested in the academic lives of the Black students with disabilities interviewed for this research. This promise of accessibility is riddled with unspoken caveats and invisible barriers that often humiliate and degrade students who must nonetheless use the programs to achieve academic success. The current policy of accommodation to individuals with identified disabilities has several shortcomings, especially when considering its application to racialized bodies and their specific needs of equity. Moreover, students may be blocked by these very programs, and many of the students expressed feeling subjugated to a "plantation mentality" and subordinated to the power structure as they tried to navigate the system. According to McKittrick (2013), "Deciphering a plantation logic, then … identifies the normalizing mechanics of the plantation, wherein Black subjugation and land exploitation go hand in hand" (p. 11). This normalization is experienced prior to even receiving supports or program access.

The "plantation mentality," as used by McKittrick in her various works, refers to the outdated and pervasive mindset that has its roots in the plantation economies during and after transatlantic slavery. This mentality rationalizes contemporary social stratification and racial hierarchy. As noted in the introductory chapter, McKittrick (2011) observes that plantation economies were defined by an uneven colonial-racial economy where Black servitude was legalized and Black placeness and constraint were sanctioned (p. 948). In this uneven colonial-racial economy, Black people were without land, home, or self-ownership. They were an inferior race under the absolute domination of white people and suffered natal alienation and social death (p. 950). While the plantation economies and their attendant mechanics are historical, the consequent psychological impact lingers today. This is the "plantation mentality" alluded to by McKittrick, where the racial power structures are normalized and reflected in the contemporary social setting, for instance, in the prison system and the prejudicial educational policies and programs that exclude the Black racial minorities and the disabled.

As a result, Black disabled students often feel undervalued and inherently inferior even as they navigate programs and systems that are said to be designed to accommodate their diverse differences. To start with, the accessibility programs and systems are mono-systemic to the extent that they overlook the inherently different and unique experiences of Black and disabled students. They may, for instance, focus on the disability and overlook the dynamics of race and how they come into play to compound their experiences. Further, accessibility programs often fail to consider the students' cultural differences (Cartledge & Kourea, 2008, p. 355). Culture is a key factor of identity that defines the individual's sense of identity. Failure to accommodate the cultural differences in the accessibility programs exacerbates the exclusion and otherness of Black and disabled students. The cultural unresponsiveness of accessibility means that Black disabled students do not obtain the much-needed accessibility, thereby hindering their academic progress. The generic accommodations inherent in the traditional accessibility programs fail to acknowledge and address the compound effects of ableism and racism experienced by Black and disabled students.

Even the access to the accessibility and accommodation programs is itself laced with racial biases, leading to disproportionate effects on the Black communities. For example, studies show that Black communities are overrepresented in special education programs due to the misdiagnosis or underdiagnosis of their needs (Blanchett, 2006; Cartledge & Kourea, 2008; Harry & Klingner, 2005). Such misplaced placements and botched diagnoses are informed by racial undertones and the plantation mentality, where the adults tasked with making the assessments and placements believe that the Black race is inherently inferior to the white race and hence have little expectations of the Black students. Annamma (2018) observes that some educational policies and programs allow the classification of students as having impairments even when they lack any notable physical impairments. These provisions may be abused by adults who seek to foster their racial privilege by negligently, inadvertently, or deliberately misdiagnosing or underdiagnosing Black students.

The plantation mentality in the accessibility programs in educational institutions also manifests in the deeply watered-down curricula and the decreased access to advanced coursework for Black students with a disability. Blanchett (2006), for instance, notes that there is a general expectation in white spaces that Black and disabled people do not have the prerequisite intellectual acumen to navigate rigorous coursework and curricula (p. 25). This practice is perhaps founded in the inherently problematic white supremacist notion that the Black race is intellectually inferior to the white race. The watered-down curriculum may insinuate that Black and disabled students are intellectually and cognitively inferior. Inevitably, the exposure to watered-down and overly simplified coursework fails to provide the intellectual stimulation required to propel Black disabled students to academic excellence.

In the university environment, disability has historically been defined as whatever educational institutions—a group including not simply teachers but also administrators and policymakers—"need" it to be to ensure the maintenance and "invisibility" of normalcy. The question now becomes: What do educational institutions need disability to be? This question is challenging and provocative as it predicates "disability" as something that requires definition not only for those categorized under its rubric but also, and in particular, for educators (teachers, administrators, and educational policymakers) who "need" it to "be" something. If one assumes these institutions to have power, this question suggests that this power is dependent—to some degree at least—upon the definition of disability in the pedagogical environments under their control. Ferri and Connor (2006) argue that the need for institutions to define disability reflects the importance of classrooms as, in Bhabha's (1994) words, "innovative sites of collaboration, and contestation, in the act of defining society itself" (Bhabha, 1994, p. 2). Ferri and Connor (2006) suggest:

> One of the socializing functions of education is that individuals come to know their place and that of their peers. In this way, education institutions, through their various sorting mechanisms, can be thought of as a colonizing force. ... Once separated into different spaces, students are socialized into an us/them binary that reaffirms culturally defined differences or "markings" such as Blackness or disability. (p. 129)

For instance, the enduring power of the medical model of disability in our culture demonstrates the need to develop and promote alternative models in the public arena. Critical disability studies, I argue, is important to the development of alternative models of disability. It is easy to conceive of people with disabilities as "other"; but it is more challenging to situate ourselves within the field of disability.

The 12 students who participated in this research presented several types of disabilities, with the majority being "hidden" or "invisible." The majority of the "invisible disabilities" were classified as learning disabilities by Accessibility Services when they made their determination about students' eligibility for benefits. An examination of the students' particular disability, their experiences with diagnosis and testing, and the accommodations afforded for their academic needs is outside the scope of this investigation; rather, I focus on the Black disabled students' interactions with their peers, professors, advisors, and service providers to lend insight into the meaning of the production of marginality as part of the normal workings of the university.

The routine practices that grant accommodations are often disconnected from the actual student performance or experience in the classroom. The task of administration is to assess and approve accommodation needs as efficiently as possible and within policy guidelines. The Accessibility Services office is "helping" students in the spirit of the university discourse of inclusivity, but what they are also doing is "helping" according to their bureaucratic policies—and they "help" only according to their own conception of disability. That brings us to the following question: *Why* and *how* are students' classroom experiences disconnected from the accommodation process? Possibly this is because the university is content with participating in symbolic activities. The process of granting accommodation is primarily symbolic and a whole apparatus has been built to create the perception of accommodation based on Blackness, disability, or class.

Obstacles

The experiences of the 12 participants were analyzed separately and then contextualized to understand their intersecting identities of ethnicity and disability status. The research demonstrates that the students' "identity," though readily defined by the Accessibility Services office and their professors, is not established by outside influences and continues to be individualistic and distinctive. That is, identity construction is not a uniform process.

In addition, the commonality of experiences between the participants reflects many societal problems associated with Blackness and disability and indicates a need to revisit the issue of how the university integrates this population into the larger student body. One of the key conclusions of this research is that "identity" is not defined solely by circumstance or opinions. Another is that the current efforts of the university to address the issue of accessibility are inadequate.

The majority of the students I interviewed indicated that they had negative experiences with the administrative personnel at the Accessibility Services office. Several noted delays in the disbursement process for such financial assistance as the Ontario Bursary for Students with Disabilities (BSWD). The delays caused financial stresses or delayed the purchasing of assistive technologies for their studies. Nearly all students stated that they had encountered discrimination either regarding their Blackness, their disability, or both. Some of the comments students received bordered on outrageous and were extremely difficult to fathom happening on a twenty-first century university campus. Because many of the students had disabilities that were hidden—not readily apparent—in a class or outside of accommodation pursuits, many chose to pass and appear "normal" to the other students and faculty who were not aware of their disabilities. A number of students voiced a reluctance to take full advantage of Accessibility Services due to prejudice from the professors and teaching assistants. For example, some professors noted in classes that disabled students had an "advantage" over other students due to the accommodations afforded them to compensate for their disabilities.

For example, Denise, a second-year master's student, stated:

> One of my professors wasn't very supportive. Due to my "invisible" disability, I had to prove to them as well by showing them my documentations to prove that I have a learning disability. And after showing him my documents he told me that he doesn't believe that this class is for me.

Barry reflected on an incident where a professor asked him about a wheelchair, stating:

> Most of my professors and teaching assistants were supportive, but I had some who were not as supportive. I had a few professors who question my disability. I literally had to justify my disability to my Political Science class professor. He then asked me where is my "wheelchair" because my disability is not physical.

David reflected on his experience with a professor whose dealings with their disability affected their academic performance:

> Oftentimes I find that my identity appears as a problem, where I found myself [being] marginalized in the classrooms. One of my professors refuses to provide me with class notes and accessible class reading materials. I reported my concern to the Accessibility Services office advisor and they told me that there is nothing they could do about it and I should try and negotiate my accommodations with my professor. I also found some of the class sizes were too large (over 150 students in one classroom) and it was very difficult to meet with professors on an individual basis.

In all, these students reported experiences that could have had a detrimental impact on their self-improvement.

The obstacles faced by students with disabilities varied. Students reported that some professors were very accommodating, while others were not at all willing to accommodate disabled students. There were also problems with study materials, particularly for students with visual impairment who relied on PDF files or audio versions of textbooks; versions that were not always available. Some students, especially those in graduate programs who had to work to support themselves, cited the hurdles they faced in their work lives as particularly challenging and contributing to difficulties in the academic setting (Annable et al., 2003; Aubrecht & La Monica, 2017; Laframboise et al., 2023; Lillywhite & Wolbring, 2022; Smith, 2005).

One way this occurs is through putting students in need of Accessibility Services into the student loan nexus. Students requiring accommodations often lack an advocate who will work to facilitate ease of access, and while students are being put in a position of indebtedness, they are also in a position of subjugation. The BSWD is particularly important for Black students with disabilities because it is the only financial program in the university that facilitates access to adaptive educational services for low-income students (OHRC, 2018). However, for students to qualify and even be considered for the BSWD, students must show proof that they are "disabled enough" to receive funding from the Ontario Student Assistance Program (OSAP) to cover costs related to academic accommodation. The system makes it difficult for Black students with disabilities to gain access to services and normalizes the processes of accommodation through bureaucratic procedures in the university setting, creating a barrier for students (George et al.,

2020; Titchkosky, 2011). The general consensus from the students interviewed was that the Accessibility Services office required them to apply for OSAP. As noted by Folake, OSAP "is an 'oppressive system' by how it functions as a tool to foster the exploitation and traumatization of students."

The understanding that Folake has in relation to OSAP is based on her own experience and the way the program links loans and services. For students to obtain services through Accessibility Services, one criterion the university uses to ascertain whether a student is worthy of accommodations is whether the student is eligible to receive OSAP. The problem is that there are many factors beyond being disabled that may impact a student's ability to access OSAP funding. International students, students who have made mistakes on OSAP applications in the past, or students who have failed a credit check, declared bankruptcy, or registered for a consolidation order may not be eligible to receive OSAP (OHRC, 2018; UofT, Academic Accommodations, 2023). For these students, this element of the evaluation process can prevent access to accommodation measures. OSAP is therefore a tool that contributes to the difficulties of Black disabled students who need these programs to improve their education experience.

The paternalistic approach to accommodation is typified by Stephanie's experience when Accessibility Services insisted that she apply for OSAP prior to receiving classroom accommodations. Students' accommodations are filtered through coercive measures that force them into a financial arrangement with the provincial government. The program facilitates provincial student aid, including student loans, and the information gathered is used to determine students' eligibility for accommodation. These processes also lend themselves to the bureaucratization of disability because students must engage with OSAP. Stephanie said:

> Initially, I would say that if I wasn't strong willed, I would have been discouraged. For me, there is a lack of respect and [there is a] racial hierarchy when accessing accommodations at Accessibility Services Office and it has become institutionalized. One of the things I thought was negative was that I would have to be on OSAP in order to actually receive any accommodations from

Accessibility Services Office. I think that's ridiculous. If I didn't already apply for OSAP, that was kind of something they pushed at you first—apply for it to see if you would be eligible. I just thought that as a university they could have been a bit better at assisting me.

The university required the disabled student to apply for OSAP prior to receiving accommodations in order to be qualified for bursaries to buy assistive technologies for their studies, again asserting control over the student in almost a plantation or paternalistic manner. The attempt to control and supervise all aspects of the disabled students' lives, because they were disabled, seems to be the most plausible explanation of the requirement to register with OSAP. This has been cited by other students in a negative light as noted by Barry, who called "OSAP the 'abusive and oppressive system.'"

OSAP operates as a gatekeeping tool of power, controlling the provision of services in the university setting. Students who cannot gain access to OSAP are at a disadvantage in that they are limited in the degree of assistance they can get for their studies. This severally limits their educational experience. For Black disabled students, these problems are important because OSAP may be the only means that will enable them to survive in the university setting. Nonetheless, OSAP presents a significant barrier for students and can create several difficulties for students as they attempt to use the system to gain access to accommodations.

The OSAP morass includes a variety of traps and confusions that can make accessibility for Black disabled students difficult. Students with disabilities may not understand what they are qualified for or how much they are qualified to receive. This can make an application for funding arduous. Further, Black students with disabilities may not understand what they are eligible for because of different income measures or accommodations tied to OSAP. The potential that they could be denied access to OSAP because of previous financial mistakes, including those involving prior use of OSAP, can also place a strain on students.

For instance, some of the major specific consequences of OSAP for students with disabilities are explained by Phillips and Collins (2017):

[For students with disabilities] 40% [or higher] course load counts as full-time status. But full-time status at the University doesn't translate to full-time status. A 40% load also means less funding. There can be long wait times before the loans are approved, often held up until the required assessments arrive, and given wait time for appointments students may end up having to pay out of pocket for e.g., first or last months' rent, course materials, etc. Managing OSAP can be like having a full-time career because there is a need for constant reporting. If you change a course load, add a course, withdraw from a course, do badly in a course, need some time away for e.g. episodic disability, OSAP monitors closely and adds or subtracts payment. A low grade in a course that indicates a lack of progress or success according to OSAP triggers a requirement for a letter and explanation. If that happens twice, you can't take any more courses until you repay. Having to think about reporting at a time when health or disability related concerns are predominant is tricky to say the least yet missing the deadlines has an impact on loans and interest on loans. (pp. 9–10)

The requirement for resources can also place a strain on the student, who could be denied access to OSAP because of mistakes made in past OSAP applications or proir financial difficulty with OSAP. At the same time, the constraints placed on eligibility for OSAP make it difficult for students to gain access to the financial resources they require to successfully receive the loan. Black students with disabilities may also fail to apply for accommodations successfully precisely because they lacked access to the accommodations that would help them complete the appropriate paperwork. For example, for students to be eligible for the BSWD, they must have a documented permanent or temporary disability, be enrolled full-time or part-time, and be registered with the Accessibility Services office. They must also be eligible for OSAP (and have at least $1.00 of financial need), which allows them to tap into some non-repayable grants (Phillips & Collins, 2017; UofT, Academic Accommodations, 2023).

Students with disabilities who are eligible for OSAP can receive up to $10,000 for learning supports (e.g., computer, accessible [assistive] technology). OSAP also administers an annual $2,000 grant for full-time students with a permanent disability (Phillips & Collins, 2017; UofT, Academic Accommodations, 2023). The students who are able to navigate the bureaucratic accommodation system and qualify for OSAP and BSWD must then account for every dollar spent through constant reporting and receipts. Such surveillance can be read—or experienced by the students—as yet another form of policing the Black body.

Thus, for must students, accommodation is tied to eligibility for OSAP. They must be pre-diagnosed with a disability, and they must never have defaulted on OSAP in the past or be overdrawn (OHRC, 2018; UofT, Academic Accommodations, 2023). In addition, every five years, a disabled student must undergo another psychoeducational or learning disability assessment to continue eligibility for the BSWD and to continue to receive accommodation. In addition, students with disabilities in higher education will be denied OSAP loans if they have reached 520 weeks of eligibility, the (lifetime limit) maximum amount of funding allowed per student. According to Thomas-Long (2010), "Graduate students who depend on OSAP might not always be eligible because they might have reached their OSAP limit by the time they enter graduate [studies]" (p. 7). For students with disabilities, these requirements make it difficult to get timetable accommodations in the classroom. For this reason, it is important to understand the administrative difficulties that students may experience in the process of gaining access to resources from the university.

Accessibility Services, as noted earlier, through the university guidelines, has absolute authority to determine the eligibility, appropriateness, and necessity of academic accommodations for the student within the statutory requirements placed upon the university (UofT, 2023, p. 2). The facilitation of this bureaucratic ordering of accommodations is through the Accessibility Services office, and as noted earlier, there are additional requirements placed on top of the student's disability for access to the accommodation.

Consequently, the rights of disabled students to education are defined and "protected" not only by the law but also by policies enacted by our educational institutions, such as postsecondary institutions. In these ways, accommodations will be made to aid students with disabilities in their studies. The stated purpose of these laws and policies is to ensure that students with disabilities have the same opportunities to education as other students. However, under these laws, the most common occurrence is that the disabled student is burdened with proving that they have a disability and that a reasonable accommodation or adjustment in the teaching instruction and assessment practices of educators is both required and feasible (Fuller et al., 2009, p. 7). The coupling of eligibility with OSAP punishes those that do not conform to the required norms. Speaking to this experience, Barry said:

> I had a traumatic experience with services. For example, my advisor did not submit my paperwork to OSAP on time, so I was punished and suspended from receiving OSAP for one year. Having to deal with the bureaucratic system of the university made me fall behind in my studies. And my advisor told me that I should "try harder." I asked her, "How can I work harder when the university has not provided me with adequate accommodation?"

The notion that Barry was not succeeding because he was not "trying hard" enough rather than because he was attempting to complete the coursework without statutory accommodations demonstrates a fundamental lack of understanding of accommodations on the part of administrators and a social failure to grasp this necessity in the first place.

This fundamental lack of understanding goes beyond mere ignorance of legal requirements for accommodations and is expressed in an underlying incredulity directed at those who do not show outward manifestations of a disability. There is a social expectation that someone with a disability should look different. This contributed to Stephanie's negative experience with Accessibility Services:

> I think I had both positive and negative experiences. I am grateful for the positive ones because they really kept me going. I had a really good advisor, but when I am doing tests and exams there were some biases: they [were] not truly supporting my learning challenges [disability]. They thought I was faking it, so to speak. For example, my advisor told me I was looking "healthy today." I think initially speaking administrators assumed that I didn't have a learning disability. Ultimately, it was kind of like, "Why do you think you have a learning disability?" or, "Did someone tell you, you had a learning disability?," as opposed to me saying, "Here are my difficulties and these are the reasons why I feel this way." It didn't seem like it was true to them; it didn't seem real.

The comment "you look healthy today" and questioning the student on why she thought she had a learning disability demonstrates the social expectation that disabled students "look different," beyond any status as a racial minority.

It would be wrong to portray the common experience as uniformly negative. In fact, most indicated that several of the administrators and employees were helpful and personable. Still, the helpful hand cannot come at the expense of personal dignity. The expressed goals of accessibility and equity are at odds with the all too frequent experience of accommodation being made with an underlying tone of suspicion, meeting the statutory obligations of accommodation but with unspoken reservation and mistrust of the disabled individual. Accommodating students with disabilities is a legal obligation of the university, one required in policy, but practicing exclusion is just as common. As Titchkosky (2011) notes, "Assertions of inclusion help to normalize conceptions of those who are essentially excludable …. Essentially excludable—this is a dominant conception of disability that operates in everyday life" (p. 39).

Practices of exclusion and discrimination often appear acceptable when bolstered by lofty goals and bold statements. The claimed benevolence of Accessibility Services should not be confused with acceptance and inclusion. Acquiescence to the legal requirements of the province and university should not come at the expense of the dignity of those they serve. The expression of support for accessibility is not the same as practicing accessibility for those needing it. For example, disability is always treated as an absent present within the university environment (Titchkosky, 2011); significantly, the Accessibility Services office holds the prism through which access is filtered, interpreted, or granted.

While educational services for students with disabilities in Canada have improved in recent years, educational researchers, and commentators in the field of disability studies note that we must put a critical eye on the initiatives and supports that educational institutions have put in place to accommodate these students. One reason for this is that many of these accommodations were not developed by the educational system but, instead, were driven by legal rulings and human rights challenges (Titchkosky, 2022; Wotherspoon, 2014, p. 268).

Discrimination

Students experienced challenges when dealing with administrative personnel and university faculty to arrange accommodations for their studies. The shared experiences are similar to a subjugated individual's request for equal treatment rather than facilitation of the delivery of a common right to those who require it. They must deal with the attitude that suggests the powerful are bestowing a privilege to those deemed worthy.

Consequently, Connell (2011) argues that we need to see disability from a "southern perspective" (p. 371). That is, we need to see that most ways of thinking about disability are grounded in colonialist, privileged thought that is geographically associated with rich, northern countries and ignores the reality that the majority of the world's disabled people reside in poorer countries. There is, therefore, an alternate approach that represents the experience of the majority of the world's population.

Although I am studying the intersection of Blackness and disability in higher education, this point is interesting because it shows that there are other perspectives on how society can develop that do not stem from the learned centers of the rich and developed world. The challenges facing Black people in North America have been the focus of scholarship for a long time now. Black people and women are just two of the main categories that have come to form "identity politics," the identifying of others in terms of their marginalization and oppression. However, these frameworks of multiple identities do not always work well together. Gilroy (2001) finds that identity is often perceived as antagonistic, as cultures, ethnicities, and other categories are pitted against each other. He notes that this approach has seen a resurgence in the past decades.

The university experience for most Black disabled students is based on their status as a racial minority, one that cannot be concealed. Visceral anti-Black sentiments are a dark undertone to all aspects of life. The open skepticism about their deservedness for accommodations is intrinsically tied to expectations that they need the "advantages" of the accommodations, not that the university itself has endorsed the need for them. Black students with disabilities are discounted and dismissed rather than accommodated and accepted.

For example, Black students with disabilities who require accommodations at the graduate level often face barriers such as unmet expectations and discrimination (Annable et al., 2003; Chataika et al., 2012; Myers et al., 2014). Students with disabilities who attempt to obtain accommodation at the graduate level will face problems and extreme frustration. For disabled students to continue to receive accommodation at the graduate level, they must undergo another psychoeducational or learning disability assessment to "prove" they are worthy of accommodation. For example, Denise stated, "My accessibility advisor asked me, 'why do you need accommodation? Our records showed that you have already completed your bachelor's degree. Now that you are in graduate school, you should be able to work independently without accommodation.'"

Black disabled students who were once assessed as having a permanent learning disability and were provided support to facilitate their academic career, are expected to work independently at the graduate level because the status of "permanent disability" no longer applies to them. At this level, what was conceived as permanent now becomes a temporary disability. It is expected that once the disabled student reaches the graduate level, they are no longer in need of accommodations because the student has learned to "manage or overcome" their disability.

In considering the absurd justifications for the exclusion of Black students with disabilities, an analogy comes to mind: Imagine going into the university library and being told they do not have any accessible study rooms. Then, upon complaining that they have signs showing they indeed have accessible study rooms, being told, "Well, isn't having a sign of something better than nothing at all?" While surreal and darkly comic on one level, in terms of education institutions and the construction of the social self, such narratives teach colonized people to have an inferiority complex (Césaire, 1972). Yet, think about the meaning of this language: power here is in the hands of the administrators, while the disabled student is denied agency over their own educational future as a consequence of policies designed for the physical space.

In the face of racism and ableism, the attempted mitigating factors of accessibility only perpetuate that "abled privilege also reproduces itself based on its relationship to normalcy. [Anti-Black] racism and ableism as discursive practices form the backbone of the ... need to maintain privilege" (Pickens, 2014, p. 38). The implied superiority reinforced through the condescending attitude in the delivery of services and accommodations "as required by policy and law" is merely a means of supplementing the power structure and asserting superiority.

These students are perceived as a "threat" to educational institutions because they disrupt the notion of normalcy that is embedded in the systematic practices of disability or Accessibility Services. Disability is generally viewed as a "problem" that exists in the disabled's individual and is in need of a bureaucratic solution "in order to cure, care for, or contain [the] disability" (Titchkosky, 2011, p. 17; see also Goering, 2015; Oliver, 1996; Shakespeare & Watson, 2002). As Titchkosky (2011) notes, "Disability is taken as an (unessential) condition the individual must overcome, adjust to, or succumb to" (p. 141). It is noteworthy and clear from the student statement above that the coloniality of power and social construction of normality are crucial factors in how Accessibility Services advisors respond to the needs of students with disabilities seeking services.

The experiences of Black disabled students are indicative of the way normalcy and coloniality continue to shape educational institutions (Mignolo, 2012; Wynter, 2003). Thus, while there were rarely overt signs of prejudice toward the student from those in authority in this university, the insidiousness of this lies in the fact that this prejudice is extraordinarily difficult to resist, for it can rarely be isolated to a single obvious incident or individual. Instead, the student's statement reveals a general pattern of prejudice toward Black students with disabilities registered with this university's Accessibility Services office.

For a Black disabled student, there are stereotypes that can never be rebutted because of the context of normalcy in our society.

These students are also faced with managing the issues or stereotypes that may arise because of a social interpretation of their Blackness, which could not be separated from their experiences of disability. In this way, these students felt their presence at the university was questioned because of their combined Blackness and disability; they were left uncertain as to what played a role and when in their marginalization. Their peers oftentimes expressed or implied that they did not truly earn their spot at the university because people with their racial background usually demonstrated difficulty with understanding complex concepts. As Lorna, a third year PhD student, noted, her peers questioned if she deserved to be in the university because people like her don't understand concepts, which made her believe she had been discriminated against. She often felt the need to prove herself, and this act itself was offensive. By actively seeking to prove herself, she acted as if her existence was not good enough, and this need to justify her existence was also offensive. Likewise, Stephanie, a fourth-year undergraduate student, stated that one of her peers asked her, "How did you manage to get through this prestigious university despite people of your kind's reputation as loud, rude, ghetto, and not academically inclined"? Blackness and disability have several similarities when viewed through a societal prism.

Unfortunately, these similarities exist because they are used as tools for marginalization and shoring up the boundaries around normalcy. This marginalization separates these students from the center and forces them to justify their existence and place within the university setting. This separation is another form of social oppression that has no place in the educational system. Finally, while we can understand the reasoning underlying the need to address the multiple and complex perspectives of particular forms of oppression and marginality, we must not overlook the intersectional reality of Black disabled students' experience. This requires looking at the lived experiences of Black university students as a prelude to understanding how Blackness and disability intersect in student lives.

The characteristics of students with learning disabilities are so far from the institutional definition of normalcy that the marginalization of students with these characteristics is bound to occur. The advisors with Accessibility Services are the gatekeepers to the necessary accommodations that the participants in this research need to meet the requirements of their individual programs and the tools for their collective success in their academic endeavors, and the denial or impeding of accommodations becomes a form of punishment for refusing to conform.

Although not directly congruent to the experience of the "urbicide" referred to by McKittrick (2011) as destroying a "sense of place" or home, the Accessibility Services office should be a safe place for disabled students to thrive and work as members of the academic community. Through the plantation mentality, which requires complete capitulation and contrition, there is exile. As McKittrick (2011) notes:

> In terms of the willful destruction of a black sense of place, then, a limited conception of race, and a limited conception of the plantation prevails: Blackness is recognizably placeless and degraded and therefore justifiably without, which is not only the commonsense outcome of our analytical queries but also evidence of a myopic plantation past. (p. 594)

The students suggested that their Blackness and disability exacerbated their experiences in the university classroom and with accessibility services. Moreover, it seems there is a taken-for-granted conception of disability that operates in the university as grounds for disqualification—thus a blurring between anti-Black racism and disability—one way or another. The students' statements seem to raise the question of who belongs.

I argue that the conception of disability reflects the popular perception that says disability is localized in an individual and, at the same time, is disrupted by how the student's called attention to their "shortcoming" regarding ability. The measure of this "shortcoming" was normalcy: defining disability while—in the process—obscuring itself from perception. Nonetheless, the reality of the existence of this shortcoming necessitates our "decloaking" normalcy and shifting the social location of disability from the stigmatized individual to the larger society that is engaged in constructing the condition.

In addition, many of the students expressed concern about the issues of power and discrimination implicated in the learning assessment tests. It cannot be denied that medical science and technology have contributed significantly to the well-being and achievement of students with disabilities, ranging from mobility to adaptive technologies for those with visual or auditory disabilities.

At the same time, however, critics have argued that assigning "medical meaning to disability" results in treating "the person with the condition rather than 'treating' the social processes and policies that constrict disabled students' lives" (Linton, 1998, p. 11). As this criticism assumes, the concept of "disability" has meaning in popular society primarily in medical terms. While this meaning would seem to be clear and unqualified, in reality it is a construction that is flawed by social biases:

> The term disability, as it has been used in general parlance, appears to signify something material and concrete, a physical or psychological condition, considered to have predominantly medical significance. Yet, it is an arbitrary definition, used erratically ... by professionals who lay claim to naming such phenomena. (Linton, 1998, p. 11)

The vague and arbitrary boundaries of the concept are significant. The power to classify someone as possessing a disability represents considerable social authority. Regardless of whether the student actually possesses a disability, or the nature of the disability, the labeling as such, it may be argued, has been characterized by a long history of discrimination. This is particularly the case in the field of education, where being assessed as having a disability has resulted, until very recently, in one's being separated from the general student population, with all of the negative emotional and social impacts stemming from this marginalization (Middleton, 1999, p. 13). Indeed, many studies have found that students assessed as possessing disabilities have not only noted differences in their teaching environment but also a general dismissal of their intellectual abilities and needs by the education establishment.

Acknowledging the everyday reality of our lived experiences of anti-Blackness and anti-Black racism, in *Black Skin, White Masks*, Frantz Fanon (1967) famously writes, "O my body, make of me always a [wo]man who questions!" (p. 232). A similar issue is noted by Simone Browne (2015) in "On the Surveillance of Blackness":

> Surveillance is nothing new to Black folks. It is the fact of anti-Blackness [in the education institutions] .... Under these conditions of terror and the violent regulation of Blackness by way of surveillance, the inequities between those

who were watched over and those who did the watching are revealed. The violence of this cumulative gaze continues in the post-slavery era ... when enactments of surveillance reify boundaries along racial lines, thereby reifying race [Blackness], and where the outcome of this is often discriminatory and violent treatment. Of course, this is not the entire story of surveillance, but it is a part that often escapes notice. (pp. 8)

Reflecting on my own personal experiences as a Black man and the experiences of the students who participated in this research, I feel Fanon's (1967) claim about how his body makes him a man who always questions. These questions arise when the body is met by the gaze of the other. Fanon also "prays" to his body; he prays for those questions that arise when the gaze of others makes one into a question, but he comes to question *that* he has been made questionable by the gaze of others. I question what harm is done by accommodating Black students with disabilities so that they are able to perform alongside, or even on the margins to, students who are not disabled.

I ask why it is that I, as a Black man, would require a watchful eye; why school policy related to security would change, thus removing my access to academic accommodations. These are personal questions. However, reflecting on the findings of this research, it would appear that others are asking the same questions. Personal experience as marginalized people contributes to our understanding of the perceptions the world has about a Black person. The evidence that backs it up is made clear in the way we must prove our disability as though accommodations are things all Black students desire. In reflecting upon Browne's (2015) ideas about the surveillance of Black men, I consider my own experiences of when my own university would watch to make sure I was working and not sleeping. It is difficult to imagine what kind of damage the school believed I could do—but I suspect the chair was thinking that far ahead.

According to Titchkosky (2007), the fact that educational institutions have decided what is in the best interest of the disabled body—through being arbiters of the interests of privilege operating in the guise of the collective—allows us to understand why "vulnerability" is such a semiotically-loaded term in our culture (p. 7). She notes how "vulnerable is a term that can allow Blackness ... and disablement to intermingle ... so that people do not have to imagine how the intersections of some social differences are made to appear natural" (p. 4).

Thus, these differences, and the attendant vulnerability, are made to appear natural through what Sara Ahmed (2007) refers to as "habit worlds" (p. 156). Ahmed argues that social institutions serve as orientation devices that enable public spaces to "take shape by being orientated around some bodies, more than others" (p. 157). Her contention that public spaces in our culture are constituted around "whiteness" and "white bodies" speak directly to both Bell's (2003) and Titchkosky's (2007) discussions of "vulnerability." These cultural texts reflect the "habit worlds" of our society, which reinforce the meaning of "vulnerability" for Black students—that public spaces are not for us.

If, as Ahmed (2007) states, "institutions provide collective or public space" (p. 157), how do we interpret the meaning of public spaces in Canada when Black students feel "vulnerable" to anti-Black racism, surveillance, harassment, and structural violence and feel blocked by barriers? Structural violence is the manifestation of violence that corresponds to the systematic ways institutions and social structures control and exploit populations. This violence is particularly insidious for the way it restricts individual agency as a source of resistance. By manifesting itself in a systematic fashion through a number of large social structures, it renders all those who are part of the structure complicit in the violence. Other scholars have shown that knowledge and education are the most effective tools for dealing with oppression. To understand this ontological marginalization and erasure, we need to understand how they are dependent upon the fact that institutional operations are obscured. That is, disability is made to seem like a tragic impairment and a non-viable status within institutions that construct some member's privilege as "natural."

One of the most promising paths of resistance to this is to reveal the artifice underlying this construction. In other words, "treat disability [and Blackness] as an interpretive issue" (Titchkosky, 2007, p. 9). Since it is in our collective interests to understand and appreciate Blackness and disability, strategies to disrupt the "habit worlds" of racist and ableist discourses can serve the common good by challenging the institutional power structure. Indeed, the success of this strategy can be seen in the counternarratives explored by Bell (2003)—where the academic communities take it upon themselves to resist the colonizing power of hegemonic institutional power. Critics in the field of education note that educational institutions have long been used by hegemonic power in societies to perpetuate colonial and Eurocentric values and standards that reproduce that power.

A significant majority of the students noted instances of racism in their educational experience comingled with their experiences as disabled students seeking accommodations through Accessibility Services. Paige shared an insight common to many in this research: "So-called visible minorities, we are definitely the students that are expected not to succeed." Some students sense a pervasive silent conspiracy of low expectations in the community. As Sarah, a woman in a male-dominated field of the sciences, stated: "[I felt like] people are watching and expecting me to fail." A more explicit complaint is related by Kimberly, regarding a research paper she was proposing for a graduate level sociology course: "Your race, your Blackness—which is vast in terms of how it plays out—does play a role in an academic institution because it is similar to the system you have any other institution."

This theme of Blackness being treated as an invitation to lower expectations was repeated in the interviews when I asked, "Do you experience Blackness and disability playing out at the University of Toronto in any other ways, or ways you haven't mentioned yet?" Participants observed that the underestimation of abilities and the assumption of not being able to achieve at the same level as non-Black students was either stated overtly or implied through the conduct of the professors. The conduct demonstrating lowered expectations was implied in most instances by not calling for their input during class discussions or not calling on them to answer questions.

This quiet racism of lowered expectations—a form of discrimination against students utilizing accommodations through Accessibility Services—needs to be juxtaposed to the perceived advantage many assume students with disabilities receive when they are given more time complete assignment or write exams, alternate test locations, or other modifications. The university follows the Ontario Human

Rights Commission's guidelines on educational accommodations by stating: "An appropriate accommodation at the post-secondary level would enable a student to successfully meet the essential requirements of the program, with no alteration in standards or outcomes" (UofT, 2023, p. 1). I argue that the important part of this statement with regards to students is the phrase "no alterations in standards or outcomes." It became abundantly clear from the interviews that there were increased expectations in terms of ability to perform and an unwillingness to provide further assistance to the students outside the classroom.

The impression is that the professors think it is easier to take the exams with accommodations, not that the students perform at a higher level. Stephanie related a similar impression, noting:

> I have to prove over and over again that I am truly intelligent enough to be a university student, or they look at you, as "I don't know if you'll work hard enough," when I have to write my test or exam at the test center. There is that negative connotation of how the professors or teaching assistants would give you a lower grade as opposed to the general class. It's how they treat you, students with a disability, not necessarily the words that they are saying. It just, that kind of sounds like the "others" as opposed to just a student.

Black disabled students in university feel that they not only have to justify their intelligence from a racial perspective but also that their disability may compromise their ability to add value to classroom discourse.

The Colonial Vestiges of Education

The education system can have negative implications for the self-worth and identity of students with disabilities since it privileges non-disability as the normative condition through its structure and curriculum. I draw on scholarly works in education on the construction of normalcy in the context of corporate and colonial power to describe how this function is analogous to the oppressive role of Canadian education for students with disabilities. However, if we critically examine the concept of "normal" in Western culture, we can understand Homi Bhabha's (1994) analysis in *The Location of Culture*. According to Bhabha:

> The great connective narratives of capitalism and class drive the engines of social reproduction, but do not, in themselves, provide a foundational frame for those modes of social identification and political affect that form around issues of sexuality, race, ... the lifeworld of refugees or migrants, [disability or Blackness]. (p. 6)

While Bhabha's (1994) view suggests that social reproduction in our society is driven by capitalism and class, it is critical to acknowledge the existence of locations of culture beyond even these forces. Bhabha's argument has points of theoretical overlap with the assertion of Ferri and Connor (2006) that the modern classroom is not only a powerful site for the social reproduction of normalizing methodologies of knowledge in our society but that it is also a key point of contention between inclusionary and exclusionary discourses.

Still, it is important to recognize that some individuals in the academic community of people with disabilities seek to emphasize difference—probably in much the same way as many Black students seek to emphasize difference as a means of representing their identity. The written policies regarding disability are completely silent on the issue of racial minority status. The plainly stated university policy on disability services says:

> The University is committed to developing an accessible learning environment that provides reasonable accommodations to enable students with disabilities to meet the essential academic requirements of the University's courses and programs. (UofT, 2023, p. 1)

The policy goes on to claim that it will ensure that these accommodations for accessibility are an implementation of the requirements proposed by the Ontario Human Rights Code, stating, "Academic accommodations for students with disabilities are provided in accordance with the statutory duty arising from the Ontario Human Rights Code" (UofT, 2023, p. 1). The acceptance of the duty to provide accommodations for disabled students is irrespective of race, color, or ethnicity and does provide an extensive grievance procedure in the advent that someone experiences discrimination based upon their status. In other words, the policy of accommodation by the university holds true irrespective of the disabled students' Blackness.

However, that is not the common experience of the students interviewed for this research. They noted an underlying tone of racial discrimination, not in the form of a denial of requisite services, but through the softer, more covert means of perpetuating the plantation mentality and condescension associated with the power structures involved. The students were not directly questioned about the effect of their racial minority status by the Accessibility Services office. My second interview question asked: "What has accessing accommodation been like for you?" While this open-ended question deliberately removed race from the question, the answers showed a common experience of racial impact on the services provided. Saga noted, in direct terms:

> My advisor at Accessibility Services Office knew that I have a disability, and my "disability" is invisible. I have a learning disability, what we now call "invisible" disability. However, I can't remove my Blackness, but I can remove my disability. What is a "normal" person, or what do we expect a disabled person to look like? Are we not human beings anyway? Although I often ask myself, "Who am I?" If you are a Black person and have a label, it will have an impact on you for the rest of your life and can prevent you from fully participating in society e.g., even getting a job and this label criminalizes you.

His answer raises other issues to be explored later, but the inseparable aspect of him being a racial minority features prominently in it. The attitude that his status of disability, although "invisible," is a deviation from the "normal" is concurrent with this visible outward appearance. He is different from other disabled students seeking services, and it is as plain as the color on his face.

This is concisely relayed by Zaine when she states, "I had come to the realization that due to my Blackness I am judged, with or without a disability." Again, this response is to my question about accessing accommodations—her response highlights the unfortunate prejudice stemming from the feeling of being judged. Notably, it is the responsibility of Accessibility Services to "judge" the students on their need for accommodations; this seems reasonable in light of the simple fact that these accommodations are only available to students that require them because of a disability. It is clearly stated in the university policy that it is the duty of Accessibility Services to carefully scrutinize each application for accommodations. The University of Toronto has an Accessibility Services office on each campus to assist students and faculty with academic accommodations. The role of these offices is to:

> Review the student's medical documentation on a confidential basis; Verify the student's disability on behalf of the University; Determine with the student based on the documentation provided whether accommodations are required and, if so, what accommodations would be effective and act as a resource for faculty in assisting with the implementation of accommodations in the classroom. (UofT, 2023, p. 1)

It is expected that Accessibility Services will carefully review each application; however, it is clearly stated that no person should be refused accommodations because of biases to their race, class, etc.

The plantation mentality is evident in several experiences of the Black disabled students interviewed. For example, when the validity of the student's disability is challenged or when accommodations that would support equity for the student are held back from the student, with the student having to prove that they should be given accommodations. The university is controlling Black disabled students by questioning their needs, which in turn has an impact on the students themselves, leading them to either question their own validity or lose faith that the university system is a place where they belong—possibly both.

The university agrees that they will provide accommodations and will even state in forms and documents what these accommodations are. However, students must be prepared to constantly prove that they require these accommodations. This approach to the learning environment reinforces the plantation mentality as the student continues to see the classroom experience as one where access to each element that would support their equitable treatment is controlled. In the face of this, they must also defend their position that their different abilities make access a requirement.

In questioning the veracity of their disability after it has been conclusively established according to the medico-bureaucratic requirements, overlaid is an additional requirement designed to place dominion and control over the disabled students through the requirement to register with OSAP. I have shown that although these efforts in most cases may not be intentional and purposeful, the subjugation of Black disabled students does occur as a matter of the bureaucratic policies and practice due to the inherent prejudices that are still present in the university and in society. The bold statement that "all may share the same level of access to opportunities" (UofT, 2023, p. 2) should have a caveat that accommodations are provided within societal expectation of the conduct of Black students.

Stigmatization

A recurring theme of the participants' university experience was the negative labeling associated with their Blackness or disability. Paige spoke to how she was able to keep going in the face of this labeling:

> Knowing myself, and basically, not allowing barriers that arose while I was going through my university experience—not allowing them to block me or to stop me from, you know, experiencing or attaining what it was that I wanted to attain. Ignoring some of the stigma, some of the snobbery that existed.

Paige related that the university continues to be a site of barriers for students with disabilities. These barriers, which can include structural barriers to accessing accommodations, seemed to signify systemic barriers to students such as herself. She felt as though even seeking accommodations for her disability victimized her because she was often forced to place herself in a vulnerable position and plead for these accommodations. Paige was unable to distinguish whether her negative experiences in accessing accommodation were due to her race, disability, or both.

This student also described seeking help from Accessibility Services as placing a "stigma" upon her academic career. The reoccurring theme of stigmatization in connection to the use of Accessibility Services, and the accommodations afforded though this, is found in many of the interviews. After all, while there may be legislation or university protocol for university accessibility for students with disabilities, and students with disabilities may represent a minimum portion of the student population, barriers to access remain the norm as opposed to the exception within the wider university environment. If students with disabilities feel they are not welcome in the university environment, is it not logical that many would prefer to stay away from Accessibility Services and avoid the energy drain of continually overcoming and/or improvising around structural barriers?

At the same time, some professors demonstrate that they do not appreciate the purpose of the modified testing or curriculum conditions. David noted:

> I asked the professor if it was possible for me to meet with him to discuss my grade. He told me that there is no need for that ... This stigma can also inform my identity and academic achievement.

David's concern is that he will be perceived as not properly earning his academic achievements and his identity will be tainted forever.

Low (1996) analyzed the identity development of disabled university students and found that it is a three-part negotiation of their disability identity, their non-disability identity, and their physical environment. This ongoing negotiation in the context of attempting to fit in as "normal" or "mainstream" is of particular concern to students with "visible" disabilities. In an environment where the potential for stigma thrives, some students do not want to draw attention to themselves any more than they already have. Christine said:

> I need to take an elevator because I have trouble going up the stairs and my knees give out. I ask someone who works in the building [at U of T], "Where is the elevator?" and then she sent me into a wild goose chase. I feel like she just looked at me, and thought, "What do you need an elevator for?" And she sent me to the stairs (giggling). And so, I look at them anyways because at that point I'm just frustrated. At that moment, I had to take out my little stick. But, I was still having difficulty accepting using the stick. The stick, it makes me feel worse because the other students always look at me with pity. The

stick had a complex range of symbolisms for me and society in general. You know, I don't like using it. I think everyone be looking at me. But for a little thing it is sure useful. I forced myself, but there is always this little fear in me, "Please don't give out. Please don't give out. Please legs get me up the stairs." It's little things like that. It's just humiliating.

Rather than continue the search for the elevator and subject herself to further insult, Christine chose to suffer the pain of using the stairs. Given my work in critical disability studies and issues of stigma and marginality, I am struck not only by the student's recognition of how her use of the stick would lead people to label her as a student with a disability—a label that she clearly resisted—but also how she used the stick as a means of resisting this foreclosure and "troubling people." In a sense, the student's stick—this "little thing"—can be considered a "prop" in her performance of disability. Like any prop in a stage or film production, its meaning derives almost entirely from its usage by characters. In this case, the student seemed to be aware of how her disability (and possibly gender or Blackness) contributed to her social making. In this context, she made use of the stick as a device to mitigate this making. In this highly self-aware performance, the student seemed to acknowledge how the stick "tagged" her as a student with a disability; a process that could result in yet another layer of social oppression and stigma. However, what was remarkable about this student's use of the stick as a prop in her performance of disability was that—I would argue—she used it as a part of an improvised strategy to not trouble people, resisting the reductionist oppressive means by which society often "reduces" individuals with disabilities to a "single attribute" (Garland-Thomson, 1997, p. 12).

The term's "performance" and "prop" in this discussion should not be interpreted as implying bad faith or an absence of legitimacy in any way. Rather, as explained earlier in the book, these terms speak to our roles as "social actors" and—from a theoretical perspective—to the theory of performative identity as presented by theorists such as Judith Butler. While the arguments made by Butler (1997) and Young (2007) that performances of identity are required by hegemonic authority as sources of legitimacy and power are well-founded, neither critic regards this as the limit of performance. For both critics—writing with regard to the performance of disability and Blackness, respectively—performance can also be deployed as a mode of resistance by social actors. While the student knew full well that the stick—an integral prop in her performance—was a well-known social marker of disability that served to identify her, she nonetheless deployed it in such a way as to resist reductionism and assert her social authority as a Black female student worthy of recognition. She used the stick as an assertion of presence and a means of overriding her "invisibility." Moreover, like any good actor, the student in her performance was highly cognizant of how her performance was being "read" by her intended audience. The student's self-awareness of her performance is made evident by her clear ambivalence in using the stick.

Against this backdrop, I argue that many Black students with disabilities are—reflective of Christine's statement above—using their performances of disability as improvised strategies of resistance to this social production of marginality and/or labeling. I would argue that Christine's anecdote illustrates the complex double-bind confronting students with disabilities—the pervasiveness of social stigma and marginalization of individuals with disabilities leaves few avenues to self-identification that are not oppressive, yet avoiding self-identification can be complicit in that same hegemonic and discriminatory order.

Barry used "pride" to overcome the stigma of disability and racism when he stated, "I am proud to be a Black disabled man." Many of the other participants, on the other hand, chose to alleviate the stigma of being disabled by enduring physical pain in an effort to hide it. Christine endured pain to climb a flight of stairs to avoid the humiliation of being sent the wrong way by a student aid when seeking an elevator rather than be further stigmatized as disabled. Recall that she stated: "I look at them anyways because at that point I'm just frustrated. I forced myself but there is always this little fear in me. Please don't give out. Please don't give out. Please legs get me up the stairs." In doing so, she separated herself from herself to deal with stigma. Similarly, Folake endured severe back pain to avoid the stigma of disability, or worse, of faking a disability: "If I experience pain during class time, I still forced myself to school. I am afraid that my professors would think that I am faking my illnesses."

In negotiating their identity, the students are attempting to avoid further stigmatization. Folake clearly articulated that "being Black and disabled there is this stigma that we're not smart enough." As Fanon (1967) relates, Black people will have to work twice as hard to prove to society that they are in fact as intelligent as their white peers.

The students noted that receiving accommodations from Accessibility Services can be challenging, and even traumatic, sometimes both emotionally and organizationally. Thus, there is an alternation between a disability being seen as a problem that can be "fixed" or being viewed with contempt as an irritant to those who must contend with their administrative duties to render accommodations for eligible students. This seemingly uncompassionate attitude toward individuals with disabilities is not unique to the university:

> There is nothing new; disability is a problem, and it is one of the many problems' sociologists have studied, for some time. Involuntary deviance, stigmatized master status, management of a spoiled identity, passing, coping, etc., are some of the most systematic representations of disability as a problem produced by sociologists. I agree there is nothing new about treating disability as a problem. Manifestations of the problem of disability and even institutional processes of its amelioration and control are things which sociologists have studied for many years. (Titchkosky & Michalko, 2009, p. 40)

The stigmatization of their identity because of a disability is one reason many of the students choose to delay or forgo the accommodations required for them to participate in all aspects of university education.

The public knowledge of confidential information regarding disability is among the stigmatizing aspects of using accommodations. At a minimum, it is impossible to keep secret that a student is taking advantage of alternative testing venues. As Folake laments:

> I was stigmatized and devalued for contributing to my undergraduate class discussions when my classmate rudely interrupted me. He asked, "What type of disability do you have?" And the professor commented by telling me another student (white) had something more important to say. Clearly, this suggests that I am intellectually inferior. And I dropped the course because

I realized I wasn't welcome in it. Being Black and disabled there is this stigma that we're not smart enough.

The accessing of accommodations is not viewed as a right for students in need, but a potential source of embarrassment. Denise, a single mother and graduate student, says:

> I found that most people including the accessibility advisors would say, "If you need accommodations, why are you here? Why not go to a community college?" That was one of their arguments to deter me from even doing an undergrad degree. And layered-on top of that was the fact that I was a single mother. So, in their eyes as a student with a disability and a single mother, it was too hard for me to develop critical and analytical thought. So why not just save the government's money and just go to a community college because that would be better. If I tried to attain a bachelor's degree, it is just going to take too long. It's a waste of time. It was traumatizing. It was stigmatizing, and it was always very embarrassing. One of the greatest anxieties you have is about being looked at as a Black student. I'm a mom and a student with a disability so now if I need help, how do I approach my professor? So that my professor doesn't look down at me and say, "Another disability student" because it always felt as if I was begging for accommodations that they said was part of my right as a student—to attain help.

The reluctance to access accommodations is typified by Zaine, who spoke to her reluctance to register with the Accessibility Services office until her last year as an undergraduate:

> It wasn't until my final undergraduate year of university that I even considered registering with Accessibility Services Office, due to the stigma that is often attached to persons with disabilities. I finally found the courage to register to receive accommodations in spite of the stigma because I had come to the realization that, due to my Blackness, I am judged, with or without a disability.

When attempting to navigate their disability, the fear of stigmatization of their disability identity brought about an internal conflict of inaction and they passed up needed accommodations or assistance for fear of diminishing their sense of self, academic or otherwise.

The responses of the students in relation to their identity stand in stark contrast to their personal assessments of their character. Where the outside world sees them as advantaged by the accommodations and having an easier path to academic success, they introspectively note a struggle against the stigma associated with their disability and often inadequate efforts by the university to accommodate. While it is prescribed by the legislative code and university rules that discrimination and segregation are not to be tolerated, their reality is a campus experience where these mandated ideals are not yet realized, and the institutions that profess to assist them have fallen far short in their efforts. This, of course, has consequences for how people conceive of themselves and forge their racial identities.

In many interviews, the students noted that their "disabilities" were "invisible," but their socially marked "Blackness" was an inescapable influence upon their experience at the university and in social settings. The interdependence that is central to the intersectional analysis cannot be viewed without first examining the individual characteristics and components of the Black disabled students' experiences.

For example, Saga, responding to a question regarding experiences as a Black disabled student at the University of Toronto, said, "I ain't disabled. I am already struggling with stigma attached to my Blackness and the whole concept of 'identity politics.' And so, I think of the term 'disability' as being ableist and another convenient way of categorizing and stigmatizing individuals based on their different learning needs."

It is interesting to note that the student chose to use the word "stigma" when discussing his Blackness and stigmatizing with regards to his disability. He cited "identity politics" and "convenient way[s] of categorizing" with regards to the issues of Blackness and disability, two interpretations of outside views on his identity. As Goffman (1967) argues, our "face," the public identity we project, is "self-delineated." We perform or enact it "in terms of approved social attributes" (p. 5) but with an interest in avoiding stigma. To this end, it is necessary that the individual "passing" be highly aware of social expectations in order to play against them. Of greater importance, Saga firmly refused to self-identify as disabled; he was, he insisted, a student that learned differently and required some special conditions to conform to the "normal" requirements of the class.

For the disabled, an element of the stigma that they experience when seeking accommodation is the feeling that we are inhibiting the optimal intellectual growth of the class by requiring services. The Foucault (1995) story "Harrison Burgereon" takes place in a society where rather than accommodating the requirements of people with different needs, they use implements as a way of disabling people. The focus of the story is on creating equality by disability. Restricting or modifying the abilities of others would be disruptive to society in unacceptable ways, but in this story, it is how the government seeks to create an equal society.

This story is a reflection on the fears that lay latent in the classroom and create stigma. They are based on the perception that students who are disabled can hold back students who are not. This reflects Wynter's (2003) discussion of colonialism in institutions and how it informs the design of their protocols. There is a paternalistic element in the way institutions manage disability by developing rules for handling the disabled. The power held by those who are not Black or disabled is maintained by having a policy in place that requires the disabled to prove the degree of their disability if they want to receive accommodations to balance out and make equal the conditions for performance, learning, housing, and so on.

Titchkosky's (2000) observation points to the implication that while disability is defined discursively by the "official text producers" of a society, this representational frame is nonetheless distinct from the real lives of people with disabilities. As Titchkosky notes with regard to the definition of disability in the medical/sociological context, "Medicine studies pathology, sociologists study deviance, and both begin with a similar conception of the disabled body—the condition of having, and thus being, a problem" (p. 208). While medical and sociological thought may define disability as a discursive project, as Titchkosky notes, this perspective has "real consequences for real people" (p. 208).

Moreover, disability is investigated from the perspective that disabled people are "problem people," and society must work with the disabled to overcome their troubles. The implication of this is that the disabled bring with them shortcomings that must be dealt with if a disabled person is brought into a work, education, or other social institution setting. Disability is therefore a social problem that extends beyond the disabled individual and will have implications for people who remain in the social sphere of the disabled. From an administrative standpoint, this can mean specific accommodations for the disabled; however, these accommodations further support the notion of the disabled being a problem requiring solutions rather than supporting the empowerment of the disabled student.

While the processes of stigmatization functions to connect individuals with "discrediting" attributes, it is important to note that this is a definitional process related to the fixed identity categories discussed above. As we have seen, identity categories are produced by regulatory authorities and have historically informed social and educational practices with regard to both Black and disabled people. These categories, characterized by their essentialism, obscure the complex lived identities of Black disabled persons who refuse to fit within the imposed binaries of our society's institutional powers. Critical Black and disability studies penetrate the cracks and gaps in these categories and allow for a more accurate, and fundamentally emancipatory, approach to identity politics for our education communities.

As Goffman (1963), one of the early scholars writing on stigmatization as a sociological phenomenon, observes, calling them "normal" or "stigmatized" does not describe people as concrete beings. It does not capture the full expression and realization of lived lives. Instead, it gives "perspectives" that are generated in "social situations." Nonetheless, despite the goals of the accessibility program and the legislation and mandates to aid students, there is a palpable scepticism about their worthiness and intellectual parity with able students and those who are not racial minorities.

The use of Accessibility Services and the organization of accommodations for Black disabled students at the University of Toronto, as demonstrated, are a right to be enjoyed by all Canadians with disabilities, regardless of social, ethic, and economic status. It is a universal requirement of the postsecondary educational system and one of the fundamental rights outlined in the Ontario Human Rights Code (UofT, 2023). There is no question that all eligible students should receive needed services without reservation or resentment. It is unambiguous in the statement of the university's policy and the law of the province.

However, in its practical application, many of society's shortcomings in terms of racial bias, distrust of racial minorities, and intrinsic discrimination by the able against the disabled are manifested. In the interviews with Black students with disabilities, it was indicated repeatedly that despite lofty elite statements to the contrary, a plantation mentality of wanting to provide assistance while also maintaining control of this segment of the population shines through the officially egalitarian policy.

Opinions regarding Accessibility Services are varied, and not all students felt that it disregarded them or that it is a necessary evil; there were a number of students who felt the system was not adverse to their Blackness and that it did not serve as a means of "exploitation, or control." Some students expressed that they had positive encounters with Accessibility Services and felt that they were helpful in obtaining accommodations for their particular needs. For example, Sarah enthusiastically shared:

> It's interesting. For me it wasn't stressful. I think I am organized and detail oriented. I'm not struggling with a physical disability or illness. I know students who fit that side of the spectrum and Accessibility Services Office hasn't been effective for them. All I needed them to do was arrange my tests, and potentially give extensions when needed. Given that those were the supports I needed, it was sufficient. I needed to take exams in my own private space. I would not have made it through university without those accommodations. I went from being suicidal and not in school to maintaining an 80 and above percentage throughout undergrad in the sciences.

Sarah went further, stating, "Accessibility Services Office was a life saver for me." David's experience was also positive; however, he did note some reservations, "I have had a great experience thus far accessing accommodations with Accessibility Services Office. The only issue I had is the design of the learning assessment tests. I believe the process of the learning assessment test is culturally framed."

In noting that the learning assessment test was "culturally framed," David was echoing, to a lesser degree, what the other students were seeing as well. Accessibility Services is designed to assist the majority of the student population and did not always anticipate the cultural needs of the Black student population. This sentiment was reiterated by Kimberly:

> I never felt initially that I had someone who could connect with me from more of a social-cultural level and whom I could trust. Trust in terms of the information I'm going to be sharing with the person. For example, will they see me the way I see myself, or are they going to treat me topically. My concern was about how would I be treated as a student that has accommodation needs but not under their context.

The responses are as individualistic as the students, and they vary among the students, but the general theme is that some felt the program was helpful, some felt it was controlling, and yet others felt that accommodations were a necessity if they were to get through their courses, but it meant tolerating the injustices that were sometimes dispensed to them in the name of assistance.

What seems to be integral in these experiences is that they are dependent upon the administrator with whom the students interacted when navigating the system. This is difficult for the Black disabled students because it also depends on the chances that an administrator has considered their own biases. Christine explains that she experienced both ends of the spectrum with her advisors at the Accessibility Services office:

> My first advisor (lady) at Accessibility Services office I had, she was great. I have a hard time dealing with what they call [being a] disabled student. I didn't like it. I thought of "disabled" as someone who is physically impaired. I have seizures and other health issues. I have that mentality that these are just things to be overcome and are not really disability. And I just look at it as if you are differently challenged. For example, my accessibility advisor tells me I should get over my disability.

The discretion involved in the process of determining eligibility for accommodation seemingly creates further vulnerabilities within and among these students. These vulnerabilities are specifically linked to the construction of eligibility for services inasmuch as they are linked to the construction of subject position categories into which students are typified.

Studies have suggested that for students with disabilities, "administrators sometimes react to requests by interpreting the laws arbitrarily and by setting contradictory or inequitable policies" (Wilson & Lewiecki-Wilson, 2002, p. 298). Moreover, the notion of power emerges as particularly relevant in the students' experiences with the accessibility advisor. Educational institutions are powerful conduits of hegemonic power because they not only shape how people are represented but also the very terms they can use to represent themselves. Christine noted that after she changed advisors, her experience changed:

> Accessibility Services offices need to be tailored to the needs of students. Whenever I meet with my accessibility advisor, I always leave that place traumatized. The previous advisor I had, she acts like you are just there to try to steal or you are trying to take advantage of the system. And so, every time I meet with my advisor, she is giving me a hard time. I always experience barriers to accessing accommodations for my studies. Instead of my advisor addressing my accommodations needs, she was treating me as a "problem"—now I become the problem instead of her dealing with my challenges. I had to deal with anti-Black racism, ableism, and genderism.

The research participants' experiences of the programs at Accessibility Services were directly tied to their encounters with the individual administrators involved. The first advisor Christine encountered was "great" and "helpful." However, with a new advisor, her experience changed, which she related to issues of anti-Black racism, ableism, and gender-based discrimination. This means returning to a critical notion of embodiment that redefines "ableism" as a condition of being able to articulate one's identity beyond normalizing modes of understanding (Goodley, 2014).

There are two primary avenues taken by the students to care for themselves: The first is to assuage the stigma of being Black in an environment where prejudice still exists, despite or even through the legislative and policy efforts of the provincial government and university. Second, subject to the shortcomings of the accommodating goals of the establishment, students navigate the different service organizations to mediate the impact of their disabilities on the university's treatment of their studies. The notion of caring indicates methods employed to counter the negative effects of society due to their Blackness and disability. These methods may not necessarily bring comfort to their lives; they only mitigate the negatives. In terms of their status as a racial body, these efforts would be aimed at finding a personal refuge from the racism and societal stigma.

Labeling

Acceptance of the potentially stigmatizing disability label brings it to confluence with the experience of Blackness on the university campus. Having a disability is the requirement for obtaining accommodations through Accessibility Services. These services are only available to students that are deemed eligible and therefore accept the label of "disabled." According to the university website, "[We are] committed to developing an accessible learning environment that provides reasonable accommodations to enable students with disabilities to meet the essential academic requirements of the University's courses and programs" (UofT, 2023, p. 1).

Acceptance by Accessibility Services is the threshold experience and milestone common to all of the students interviewed. It is here the power structure is most prominent because, without these accommodations, most of the students would be unable to participate in their university studies. Saga, building upon his experiences with Accessibility Services, relates a very traumatic and humiliating experience of personal subjugation:

> I had difficulty learning and the Accessibility Services office advised me to do the learning assessment test, which was very traumatizing for me. The assessment test lasted for two days, 3 hours a day. In a way, it places me in a vulnerable position. The process of getting these accommodations, it required me to go through a psychological boot camp. And this psychological boot camp also felt like I was in a psychological war zone and this process is very violent. This violence I experienced was very real! I was in that assessment room asking myself, "How can I escape this violent space? Why are they playing tricks with my brain?" I don't know, but it certainly feels that way. I really wanted to escape at this moment, "But no," I say to myself, "My academic accommodations depend on it." During the assessment process,

I had to reveal a lot to the person who administered the psychological test. I had to tell them about my personal medical history in order for them to approve my accommodations.

Saga not only had to prove his disability to Accessibility Services but also had to personally accept his disability-associated social stigma, a label that he rejected. Foucault (1994) notes, when stating the conditions of a punitive society, that there are four forms of punishment: the first is to banish or exile the offender; the second is a legal penalty of compensation or payment of damages to the injured; the third involves marking or labeling: "Expose, mark, wound, amputate, make a scar, stamp a sign on the face or the shoulder, impose an artificial and visible 'handicap,' torture—in short, seize hold of the body and inscribe upon it the marks of power" (Foucault, 1994, p. 23;); and the fourth is confinement.

The assessment process that the student must go through has implications in terms of their degree of accessibility; thus, the student internalizes the elements of the assessment as parts of their identity. The important aspects, as emphasized, are the labels as "marks of power" that remain part of the ongoing medico-bureaucratic circulation of power. Here it is exercised through acceptance of the disabled label, since, as noted by most of the students, their disability is "invisible." Other than the attaching of a label, they are indistinguishable from the able.

These assessment tests are not the true measure of the accommodation seekers individuality but a common threshold through which they all must pass and accept the authority to which they must submit. Assessment tests and the subsequent determination of eligibility for services reflect the hierarchies of power that exist within the university setting. The testing process and respective materials are replete with cultural biases, as was noted in the student interviews.

As noted earlier by David, "The only issue I had is the design of the learning assessment tests. I believe the process of the learning assessment test is culturally framed." Conformance to the dominant culture is required to access their services, and the Accessibility Services office resists incorporating the culture of the clients. This was also noted by

Denise as a lack of sensitivity to the cultural norms of the Accessibility Services clients, requiring their submission to the dominant majority cultural norms:

> It almost seems to me that if you are marginalized, you have to give in to the trauma and the violence. This is the only way to get the service. And that, to me, always felt very demeaning. Being marginalized and having to access Accessibility Services office for accommodation is traumatizing. Even though you need this help, it's traumatizing because you're consistently going in and saying, "Here is my heart, that's how it beats, it's healthy, but it does have one glitch that doesn't really beat really well. Over here on the left ventricle …" No one wants to do that. If I call for help, why don't you ask me what I need? Don't say how can I help you and then when I give you a one-way answer, don't treat me like I'm trying to hide something from you. It's my cultural influence that makes me so guarded. It's not that I'm trying to hide anything. I'm just not an open person. And then, I'm talking to people who don't look like me.

In speaking to her cultural divergence from the accepted norm and having to accept the dominant cultural aspect of revealing personal information, she noted that it "doesn't make me feel good," because she had to admit to an unfamiliar party that she needed help. It is only through the subjugation of self, an acquiescence to the dominant culture, and an acceptance of the power of the gatekeepers of statutorily mandated services and aid that she is able to access the support she needs. This is a complex process where the student can only transform into what they want to transform into if they become what the system and access to its services make them become. For the disabled student, these demands have ramifications for their identity and can result in the student changing in ways they did not intend.

As Gilroy (2009) notes in discussing the loss of humanity when confronting the dominant culture, this subservience removes cultural identity through the colonial attitudes of the ruling class:

> Struggles against racial hierarchy have contributed directly and consistently to challenging conceptions of the human. They valorised forms of humanity that were not amenable to colour-coded hierarchy and, in complicating approaches to human sameness, they refused the full, obvious force of natural differences even when they were articulated together with sex and gender.

> These struggles shaped philosophical perspectives on the fragile universals that had come into focus initially on the insurgent edges of colonial contact zones where the violence of racialized statecraft was repudiated, and cosmopolitan varieties of care took shape unexpectedly across the boundaries of culture, civilization, language, and technology. (p. 7)

The often open contempt with which some of the students were viewed in attempting to access needed services made them feel as if they were cheating the system, and unless they surrendered to the dominant culture, they felt they were not worthy of supports, nor even of their legal rights. Only through accepting the power structure were they able to gain acceptance from the Accessibility Services office.

Many students who participated in this research did not view themselves as disabled; they acknowledged a difference in learning methods, the amount of time required to complete an assignment or take a test, or a different need in terms of testing environment. The command to normalcy is shown as a dichotomy of personal perspectives and introspections, an "A" or "B" decision and demarcation, an "either/or" proposition:

> Equally as ironic, the compelling and seductive character of normalcy conceals the compelling and seductive character of the margins, and it conceals this not only from its "view" but from ours as well. Normalcy accomplishes this concealment by conceiving of marginality as a kind of "nowhere" and also as a "somewhere" where no one wants to be since it is virtually uninhabitable. From the standpoint of the centre, no one desires to inhabit a disabled body, or disabled senses or minds, since to do so is tantamount to barely living at all. The centre conceives of disability as a devalued life where its only hope for even a semblance of value is to evoke the "human spirit" and to "overcome disability," to adapt, to adjust, and to live as normally as possible. Such a conception of the relation between disability and normalcy holds out only two options for disabled people: we overcome our disabilities and are heroic or we do not and are tragic. (Titchkosky & Michalko, 2009, p. 7)

From this perspective, for many students in this research, "disability" is not a defining characteristic—or the particular trait that qualifies them for Accessibility Services is not a deviation from the "normal" but an integral aspect of their being. This sensibility is best represented by

Saga's defiant stance of the self-affirmation "I ain't disabled." There is a concept of "normalcy" contained in that statement. There is a perception that disabilities make someone different from the "normal" student population.

Even among the students, there was a varying concept of "normalcy." As noted earlier, Christine said: "I have a hard time dealing with what they call [being a] disabled student. I thought of 'disabled' as [meaning] someone who is physically impaired." While she did not accept Accessibility Services' normalcy definition, because her disability was learning-based, it offered her unique challenges in comprehension, leading her to contrast her personal experience with her grandfather's, who was blind. Christine accepts that her grandfather was disabled because that disability was visible to the outside world, and this was something that she had to overcome to navigate a "normal" world. Consider, for example, Shakespeare and Watson's (2002) discussion of studies that note how people with disabilities are often highly resistant to identifying themselves with their disabilities:

> Many disabled people do not want to see themselves as disabled, either in terms of the medical model or the social model. They downplay the significance of their impairments and seek access to a mainstream identity. ... There is also the issue of multiple identities. (pp. 20–21)

This clearly parallels the experience of the students who refuse to identify themselves by their impairments and, instead, insist upon being identified as individual human beings. In this research, the social model of disability must consider disability not only in terms of social oppression but also in its implications for the identity of those with impairment. Obviously, many impairments impact the lives of those who possess them. However, the question is: Do these impairments define their identity? Are we more than the accidents of fate that influence the pigmentation of our skin or physiological condition?

For the power structure of the administration of the Accessibility Services office, the normal procedure is that disabled students prove their need for services by reaffirming that they personally deviate from the normal and thus require access to remedial services. The requisite acknowledgment that the student is not "normal" is part of the threshold discussion of eligibility for accessibility services. Among the normalcy aspects of the common experience with Accessibility Services is the presumed need for other forms of financial assistance available to all students with or without disabilities. The university-imposed "normal" is that disabled students are thus required to apply for financial aid through OSAP to be eligible to receive accommodation.

This is another form of labeling, as noted above, but also another way to further distance the student from normalcy. As noted by Stephanie in her interview:

> One of the things I thought is negative was that I would have to be eligible for OSAP and receiving at least $1 in government loan in order to actually receive any accommodations from Accessibility Services Office. I think that's ridiculous. If I have a notable disability, I think that the university should find a way to assist me even if I'm not eligible for OSAP. I just thought that as a university they could have been a bit better at assisting me.

This conceptualization of normalcy means that the student requires accommodations and must subscribe to their personal deviation from normalcy with regards to their physical or mental acuity, but they must also subscribe to their financial deviation for normality requiring their enrollment in OSAP. Therefore, in conformance with the power structure, they are not only physically or mentally normal, but lacking financial normalcy as well.

The acceptance of this is difficult for many students who do not consider themselves disabled but able and simply requiring some accommodations for their alternate needs in learning. The additional subjugating requirement to seek personal financial assistance is just another form of labeling and marking the students, as noted earlier, as a form of punishment or incarceration.

Among the students, there is an open refusal by many to personally accept the standards of normalcy imposed upon them by the social power hierarchy. As previously noted by Kimberly: "I choose not to label myself as disabled. I do accept that I'm a Black student in the social context. The idea of being a disabled student—I do not agree with the term because I feel that everyone's learning needs or learning issues that are unique to him or her."

Kimberly offers an unequivocal denial of personal labels and deviation from normalcy, but an acceptance that she must bear these labels imposed upon her to receive the promised accommodations from Accessibility Services. The common experience for the students is that they must accept the label and the social construct of their deviation from normalcy.

However, others choose to embrace this characterization of themselves as disabled. For example, Barry embraced the label, using all the associated negative connotations as a badge of honor, showing his personal strength to overcome what society has determined as a disadvantage and hindrance to success. From this perspective, the marginalization of Blackness and disability must be understood as issues that legitimize the hierarchical system of power and privilege. The noticing of difference from the "norm" is always the making of marginality, and thus the power of normalcy is itself normalized.

It is noteworthy that the very notion of "marginality" denotes a distancing from a center, a center often characterized as normal. Thus, marginalization is the process of departure and distancing from this constructed norm and is propagated in the space between individuals but also between institutions (such as universities) and individuals. Marginalization in this sense is a social process done by people to other people. Despite this departure from normalcy, there are social and textual signifiers that seek to define students based on their categorization, surrounding the "abnormal" with various normalizing rules and regulations, which limit their activities and foreclose future educational possibilities. Such attempts at foreclosure are often hegemonic process that limit the educational possibilities signified by "Blackness" and "disability."

References

Ahmed, S. (2007). A phenomenology of whiteness. *Feminist Theory, 8*(2), 149–168.

Annable, G., Watters, C., Stienstra, D., Symanzik, A., Tully, B. L., & Stuewer, N. (2003). *Students with disabilities: Transitions from post-secondary education to work: Phase one report*. Canadian Centre on Disability Studies.

Annamma, S. (2018). *The pedagogy of pathologization: Dis/abled girls of color in the School-prison Nexus* (1st ed.). Retrieved from: https://www.routledge.com/The-Pedagogy-of-Pathologization-Disabled-Girls-of-Color-in-the-School-prison-Nexus/Annamma/p/book/9781138696907.

Aubrecht, K., & La Monica, N. (2017). (Dis)embodied disclosure in higher education: A co-constructed narrative. *Canadian Journal of Higher Education, 47*(3), 1–15.

Bell, L. A. (2003). Telling tales: What stories can teach us about racism. *Race, Ethnicity and Education, 6*(1), 3–28.

Bhabha, H. K. (1994). *The location of culture.* Routledge.

Blanchett, W. J. (2006). Disproportionate representation of African American students in special education: Acknowledging the role of white privilege and racism. *Educational Researcher, 35*(6), 24–28.

Browne, S. (2015). *Dark matters: On the surveillance of blackness.* Duke University Press.

Butler, J. (1997). Performative acts and gender constitution: An essay in phenomenology and feminist theory. In K. Conboy, N. Medina, & S. Stanbury (Eds.), *Writing on the body: Female embodiment and feminist theory* (pp. 401–417). Columbia University Press.

Cartledge, G., & Kourea, L. (2008). Culturally responsive classrooms for culturally diverse students with and at risk for disabilities. *Exceptional Children, 74*(3), 351–371.

Césaire, A. (1972). *Discourse on colonialism.* Trans. J. Pinkham. Monthly Review Press.

Chataika, T., Mckenzie, J. A., Swart, E., & Lyner-Cleophas, M. (2012). Access to education in Africa: Responding to the united nations convention on the rights of persons with disabilities. *Disability & Society, 27*(3), 385–398.

Connell, R. (2011). Southern bodies and disability: Re-thinking concepts. *Third World Quarterly, 32*(8), 1369–1381.

Fanon, F. (1967). *Black skin, white masks.* Trans. Charles Lam Markmann. Grove Press.

Ferri, B. A., & Connor, D. J. (2006). Challenging normalcy: Dis/ability, race, and the normalized classroom. In *Reading resistance: Discourses of exclusion in desegregation and inclusion debates* (pp. 127–143). Peter Lang.

Foucault, M. (1994). Subjectivity and truth. In J. Faubion (Ed.), *Ethics: Subjectivity and truth* (pp. 87–92). New Press.

Foucault, M. (1995). *Discipline and punish: The birth of the prison.* Trans. Alan Sheridan. Random House.

Fuller, M., Georgeson, J., Healy, M., Hurst, A., Kelly, K. Riddell, S., Roberts, H., & Weedon, E. (2009). *Improved disabled students' learning: Experiences and outcomes.* Routledge.

Garland-Thomson, R. (1997). *Extraordinary bodies: Figuring physical disability in American culture and literature.* Columbia University Press.

George, R. C., Maier, R., & Robson, K. (2020). Ignoring race: A comparative analysis of education policy in British Columbia and Ontario. *Race Ethnicity and Education, 23*(2), 159–179.

Gilroy, P. (2001). Joined-up politics and postcolonial melancholia. *Theory, Culture & Society, 18*(2–3), 151–167.

Gilroy, P. (2009). *Race and the right to be human*. Utrecht: Faculteit Geesteswetenschappen, Universiteit Utrecht. https://www.uu.nl/file/25347/download?token=l4P8qOH4.
Goffman, E. (1963). *Stigma: Notes on the management of a spoiled identity*. Penguin Books.
Goffman, E. (1967). *Interaction ritual: Essays on face-to-face behavior*. Anchor Books.
Goodley, D. (2014). *Dis/ability studies: Theorising disablism and ableism*. Routledge.
Goering, S. (2015). Rethinking disability: The social model of disability and chronic disease. *Current reviews in musculoskeletal medicine*, 8(2), 134–138.
Harry, B., & Klingner, J. K. (2005). *Why are so many minority students in special education?: Understanding race & disability in schools*. New York: Teachers College Pr.
Laframboise, S. J., Bailey, T., Dang, A. T., Rose, M., Zhou, Z., Berg, M. D. ... & Sinclair, K. (2023). Analysis of financial challenges faced by graduate students in Canada. *Biochemistry and Cell Biology*, 101(4), 326–360.
Lillywhite, A., & Wolbring, G. (2022). Undergraduate disabled students as knowledge producers including researchers: Perspectives of disabled students. *Education Sciences*, 12(2), 77.
Linton, S. (1998). *Claiming disability: Knowledge and identity*. New York University Press.
Low, J. (1996). Negotiating identities, negotiating environments: An interpretation of the experiences of students with disabilities. *Disability & Society*, 11(2), 235–248.
McKittrick, K. (2011). On plantations, prisons, and a black sense of place. *Social & Cultural Geography*, 12(8), 947–963.
McKittrick, K. (2013). Plantation futures. *Small Axe*, 17(3), 1–15.
Middleton, L. (1999). The social exclusion of disabled children: The role of the voluntary sector in the contract culture. *Disability & Society*, 14(1), 129–139.
Mignolo, W. D. (2012). *Local histories/global designs: Coloniality, subaltern knowledges, and border thinking*. Princeton University Press.
Myers, M., MacDonald, J. E., Jacquard, S., & McNeil, M. (2014). (Dis)ability and postsecondary education: One woman's experience. *Journal of Postsecondary Education and Disability*, 27(1), 73–87.
Oliver, M. (1996). *Understanding disability: From theory to practice*. St. Martin's Press.
Ontario Human Rights Commission. (2018). *The opportunity to succeed: Achieving barrier-free education for students with disabilities. Post-secondary education*. Retrieved from http://www.ohrc.on.ca/en/opportunity-succeed-achieving-barrier-free-education-students-disabilities/post-secondary-education.
Pickens, T. (2014). You're supposed to be a tall, handsome, fully grown white man: Theorizing race, gender, and disability in Octavia Butler's *Fledgling*. *Journal of Literary & Cultural Disability Studies*, 8(1), 33–48.
Phillips, S., & Collins, K. (2017). *Rads roads exploring the life travels of Ryerson alumni of disability studies*. Ryerson University, Disability Studies. Retrieved from https://www.ryerson.ca/disabilitystudies/about-school/alumni.html.
Shakespeare, T., & Watson, N. (2002). The social model of disability: An outdated ideology? In *Exploring theories and expanding methodologies: Where we are and where we need to go* (pp. 9–28). Emerald Group Publishing.
Smith, D. E. (2005). *Institutional ethnography: A sociology for people*. AltaMira Press.

Thomas-Long, R. (2010). *The politics of exclusion in graduate education.* Peter Lang.
Titchkosky, T. (2000). Disability studies: The old and the new. *Canadian Journal of Sociology, 25*(2), 197–224.
Titchkosky, T. (2007). *Reading and writing disability differently: The textured life of embodiment.* University of Toronto Press.
Titchkosky, T. (2011). *The question of access: Disability, space, meaning.* University of Toronto Press.
Titchkosky, T., & Michalko, R. (2009). *Rethinking normalcy: A disability studies reader.* Canadian Scholars' Press.
Titchkosky, T. (2022). University inclusion practices—Re-encountering the status quo: An interpretive approach. *Journal of Disability Studies in Education (online), 3*(1), 102–124. https://doi.org/10.1163/25888803-bja10017.
University of Toronto. (2023). *Academic accommodations.* http://www.viceprovostsudents.utoronto.ca/publicationsandpolicies/guidelines/academicaccommodation.htm.
Weber, M. (1947). *The theory of social and economic organization.* New York: The Free Press.
Wilson, J. C., & Lewiecki-Wilson, C. (2002). Constructing a third space: Disability studies, the teaching of English, and institutional transformation. In Sharon L. Snyder, et al. (Eds.), *Disability studies: Enabling the humanities* (pp. 296–307). Modern Language Association of America.
Wotherspoon, T. (2014). *The sociology of education in Canada: Critical perspectives* (4th ed.). Oxford University Press.
Wynter, S. (2003). Unsettling the coloniality of being/power/truth/freedom: Towards the human, after man, its overrepresentation—An argument. *CR: The New Centennial Review, 3*(3), 257–337.
Young, V.A. (2007). *Your average nigga: Performing race, literacy, and masculinity.* Wayne State University Press.

Part III

Confronting and Dismantling

The emboldening of anti-Blackness manifests in various ways. The subtlest form is through racial microaggressions against Black people, while the most dramatic form is in systemic forms of racism that have their roots in colonial practices. The notion of ableism equally contributes to the exclusion and otherness of the people living with disabilities. The intersection of Blackness and disability places Black disabled persons in a precarious position where they bear the brunt of both anti-Blackness and ableism sentiments. It is, therefore, imperative to confront and dismantle anti-Blackness and ableism to meaningfully address the embedded inequalities suffered by Black disabled people.

An intersection exists between race and disability as forms of marginalized identities. These result from ableism and anti-Black racism in society. Marginalized groups each have their own unique experiences, which impact how they navigate education, employment, health care, and other systems (George et al., 2020; Schalk, 2022). Douglas (2022) uses the example of how African American learners have a three-fold likelihood of being diagnosed with intellectual disabilities compared to white learners. This stems from the fact that their minority status exposes them to many social determinants of health. Harris (2021) illustrates how many Black communities live near natural gas facilities thus exposing the community to toxic emissions that eventually cause cancer. Black children living in these settings tend to have higher rates of asthma and thus disability compared to other racial groups.

The lived experiences of Black people and people with disabilities are compounded. For instance, Black people are recipients of police brutality. On top of that, the police tend to target persons with disabilities (Pickens, 2013). Douglas (2022) reports that one-third of the Black victims of police brutality also happen to be living with disabilities. In other words, ableism and racism intersect to create a double jeopardy. Furthermore, Connor et al. (2016) affirms that when Black students receive learning disability diagnoses they get worse treatment in the classroom than their white counterparts. Usually, white students in the upper and middle classes tend to have modifications and accommodation in the general classroom. However, Black students are often taken to segregated settings. That perpetuates their marginalization and worsens their lived experienced (Morgan, 2023).

Being a person of color with disabilities often requires innovativeness. For instance, in one case, a person of color had a condition that would not allow her to sit on a chair for longer than two hours (Chordiya & Protonentis, 2024). She did not have a lot of resources but decided to make the most of the situation through alternatives like not siting at all since there were no ergonomic chairs. The lack of resources thus necessitates a compromise.

Several alternative approaches may be adopted to disrupt anti-Blackness and ableism in their various manifestations. Pieterse et al. (2023) make a case for the use of counseling psychology in addressing racism and its psychological effects by increasing the awareness of the subject (p. 237). They observe that counseling psychology in the context of addressing racism has been reactive rather than proactive and assert that there is a need for it to evolve to bring about the desired change. They reason that racism and anti-Blackness are now deeply embedded in North American institutions and, therefore, there needs to be a change in the approaches to addressing it. Counseling psychology, for instance, ought to shift its focus from individual-level racism to systemic racism (Pieterse et al., 2023, p. 238). Further, they advocate for multisystemic and strengths-based approaches to counseling psychology to effectively and impactfully address the adverse effects of racism.

Various ideological components such as anti-Blackness, white supremacy, and radical capitalism interlock, translating into policies and practices that are designed to reproduce whiteness and white privilege. Therefore, addressing and dismantling these ideological components would be a solid start to confront and dismantle racism against Black people (Arday, 2018; Bratman & DeLince, 2022; Pieterse et al., 2023). The fact that counseling psychology focuses on individual-level racism and ignores structural racism is counterproductive because it legitimizes Black prejudice and white supremacy.

Storying survival is also one of the approaches that can be used to confront and dismantle anti-Blackness and ableism. Storying survival offers stories of people's experiences of surviving racial trauma to advocate for liberation, radical healing, and Black survival (Young et al., 2023, p. 276). Young et al. (2023) observe that storying survival has five interconnected components: storying influences, the mechanisms of storying survival, the contents of storying survival, context of storying survival, and the impact of storying survival. They argue that storying survival is a powerful approach because it significantly contributes to "critical consciousness, radical hope, strength and resistance, cultural self-knowledge and collectivism" among Black communities (p. 279). Pieterse et al. (2023), agree that storying survival will center the voices of Black people in the fight against racism (p. 238). In this way, Black people would apply their epistemology to their survival experiences. In a society where the adverse effects of white supremacy, racial microaggressions, and systemic racism are obscured by white privilege, narratives on the lived experiences of the survivors will undoubtedly reinforce the notion of resilience, underscore the fact that the experiences of Black people are similar, and give hope for true healing.

While the discussion of storying survival is exclusively limited to the racial exclusion of Black people in the reviewed literature, there is reason to believe that this approach may also be extended to fighting against the discrimination experienced by disabled people or, better still, the Black people living with disabilities. Gatekeeping in scholarly research publications is also fronted as one of the ways anti-Black racism may be confronted and actively dismantled. Specifically, it is argued that articles that tacitly endorse racism or that fail to confront racial inequalities should be denied the honor of publications. Alternatively, encouraging excellent research in anti-Black racism and detailing narratives on individual experiences of Black prejudice is essential.

Discrimination against Black people with disabilities may also be confronted and dismantled by reviewing course syllabi and curricular content. This is another way gatekeeping may be used to actively fight anti-Blackness. Bratman and DeLince (2022) recommended this approach following their study, which was primarily focused on teaching environmental studies and sciences (p. 194). They correctly argue that there is a need to decolonize the ESS courses, which they note are laced with white supremacy sentiment and subtle tendencies to obscure and perpetuate white privilege. One of the ways this can be done is by broadening the diversity of the authors in the course syllabi (Bratman & DeLince, 2022, p. 195). This suggestion is based on sound reasoning, which states that no one owns knowledge and that it is not the preserve of a particular race. Some of this knowledge originates from the racial minority population's traditionally overlooked and excluded experiences. Therefore, a broader representation of the traditionally excluded Black communities in the authorship of various course materials will contribute to anti-racism.

By so doing, the notion that environment movements and knowledge originate in the white race will be confronted and dismantled. The overrepresentation of white authors in course syllabi is one of the ways that white supremacy is underpinned in academia. This argument is compelling and persuasive because academia has, for the longest time, been used to perpetuate white privilege in subtle ways. Interacting with academic material from primarily white authors reinforces the notion that the white race is superior and the Black race is inferior. Against this backdrop, the argument for a review of the course content and the representation of racial minorities in the authorship of course material will help society to unlearn the problematic ideologies of anti-Blackness and white supremacy.

Joyce and Abdou (2023) also endorse this approach, reasoning that curricula, particularly the depiction of ancient African societies in secondary school history textbooks, reinforce the ideologies of anti-Blackness and racism (p. 1054). They observe that the history textbooks in Canada have hegemonic discourses in their representation of Black history. White supremacy is subtly represented as common sense and logic. The textbooks have figurative statues that inform the way society conjures the images of racial hierarchy. The effect of these figurative statues is that they normalize historical and contemporary racial inequalities and injustices. The figurative statutes, like the physical statutes, Joyce and Abdou argue (2023), shape society's perceptions and interpretation of social structures and racial power dynamics. The hegemonic discourses in the history textbooks are not accidental but are deliberate projects of white supremacist capitalist patriarchy. Therefore, since curricula are essential in shaping our understanding of history and society's perception of social structures, there is a need to review the curricular content to eliminate the problematic depiction of race and racial domination that constructs social hierarchies. The curriculum, especially on history, should appreciate the complexity of Blackness and underscore the agency of Black communities as opposed to the Black communities' entanglements of mutual indebtedness.

Another approach to confirming and dismantling discrimination against Black people with disabilities is by increasing awareness of ability profiling, racial profiling, and subtle racial microaggressions. It is noteworthy that the otherness and exclusion of Black and disabled people are so prevalent in society today. Racism, ableism, and attendant physical and symbolic violence are so prevalent today that they are often taken for granted and passed on as usual (Bratman & DeLince, 2022; Reiter & Reiter, 2020). Owing to this normalization, society, including the Black and disabled communities, becomes complicit in their systemic exclusion and profiling and the attending damage. Therefore, notions of normalcy, inclusion, and belonging should be actively challenged to achieve equality and equity (Arday, 2018, p. 145). One of the ways that this can be done is by calling out and confronting situations of racial microaggressions. Anti-racism discourses often overemphasize the blatant and obvious manifestations of racism and overlook its subtle and covert manifestations.

The most common manifestations of racism are subtle and covert microaggressions. Microaggressions are "the commonplace everyday exchanges that send demeaning and belittling messages to people of color because of their membership in a minority racial group" (Reiter & Reiter, 2019, p. 30). For instance, there may be microaggressions that depict the Black race as academically inferior, less articulate, criminal, promiscuous, less attractive, loud, angry, threatening, and pathological. Since these aggressions are so commonplace, society, including the Black community, has accepted them as usual, with some victims believing that they are inherently true. For instance, Black students are reported to drop out of school out believing they are less intellectually capable than their white peers. Therefore, to meaningfully dismantle the discrimination against Black people living with disabilities, there is a need to unlearn the tendency to normalize all manifestations of racism.

Chapter 6

Embedded Marginalization

There is much that needs to be done to address the current problems that exist at the intersection of Blackness and disability. In the case of this book, the focus is on how universities approach their treatment of students with disabilities.

I employed post-traumatic stress disorder (PTSD) as an example that helped to orient and frame understanding disability more generally, and how this orientation to disability grounds some of the research interests. For the university student, there are several disabilities that are carried into the university setting. These disabilities can require accommodation on the part of faculty and administration to ensure that the student has equal access to the preparation and growth that happens in the university setting. While I used the distinctive example of PTSD, there are several other disabilities that could have been used. PTSD contributed to the frame of this research and to my interest in the problem.

In the process of reflecting on PTSD and disability for this book, I became mindful of the metaphorical statement that people with disabilities live in the "gap" between the real and the representational.

Oddly, this "gap" kept bringing to my mind the famous London Underground warning—repeated automatically at subway stations in London, England, for years—to "Mind the Gap." There was a gap between the subway platform and the old subway cars. The voice recording of this phrase, which is featured in many British movies and TV shows, somehow encapsulated the importance of this issue for my book. People with disabilities and/or people labeled with a disability-like condition, such as PTSD, live their daily lives suspended in the gap between themselves as an "I" and the power of institutional forces pressing to define them with a label or designation. For instance, Foucault (1995) defined the term "enclosure" to better understand how social institutions would limit and separate people from one another (p. 141). With further introspection, the thought occurred to me that I cannot consider myself as an "I" totally divorced from my social condition or fixed identity categories. While I do not accept the power of institutional forces to limit or fully define me or my possibilities, at the same time I cannot ignore the very real fact that these forces define the world through which I move on a daily basis. They have, as Titchkosky (2000) noted, "real consequences for real people" (p. 208). This gap and its consequences are part of what animates the research in this book.

"I" am not defined by the diagnosis of PTSD; however, at the same time, the fact that it has troubled me and has caused no small amount of reflection shows that I cannot consider my reality in isolation from its social representation. In a sense, we all exist in a state of dynamic tension, living our daily lives in the gap between the real and the representational. What this view suggests is that we cannot ignore the fight for inclusion and equity, despite our best efforts to do just that. What is going on in the greater world regarding the definition of fixed social identities is typified by those associated with disability or PTSD.

In the classic movie *Casablanca* (Curtiz, 1942), the protagonist Rick, played by Humphrey Bogart, is often seen as representing an isolationist United States that has retreated from the fight against fascism in Europe. At one point, as Rick is debating engaging in the fight with Signor Ferrari, Sydney Greenstreet laments that in the modern world, "Isolation is no longer a practical foreign policy." In a very real sense, this statement can be seen to apply our understanding of disability in terms of living in the gap between the real and the representational. While it is at times undeniably exhausting and emotionally troubling to have to continually navigate the innumerable forces in this gap, it is worth reiterating that it also undeniable, as second wave feminism noted so aptly, that "the personal is political" (Hanisch, 2006, p. 1). This analysis has important social and political consequences, especially when connected to taken-for-granted relations of disability as a problem or when exclusion is naturalized in the processes of stigmatization.

Power is an important element of my research. Through power and control, current social paradigms can be maintained or disrupted. The approach taken by universities with regard to Black disabled students is such that the current paradigm is maintained through policies that dictate what disability means and how the individual with a disability may be handled. In my personal experience, this is handled in the university in such a way that the university maintains control over the person and their personal construction of their disability by maintaining the nature of accommodation. This is power and this is how the system is maintained—by making the disabled prove their disability. My research project interpreted what this power does to the Black disabled students who needs to deal with faculty and administrators.

This discussion reveals things I have in common with many of the students interviewed. Many of them have learning disabilities that are "invisible." Like me, several of the students have also been diagnosed with PTSD. I contend that we cannot yield ground but must contest every inch of the definitional "no-man's land": disability and PTSD are intellectual and cultural battlefields. While it is inescapable that we are represented as "problem people," especially when we refuse to admit that we are "problems," it is critically important that we not accept this classification as limiting us, or defining who we are as human beings. We live lives that interact with our disability, our Blackness, our gender, our age as fixed identity categories, engaging in performative politics in responding to these definitional categories in public spaces while retaining our sense of ourselves as "I"s that nonetheless stand apart from the performance in some respect. Thus, there are also political interests that militate on behalf of the recognition of PTSD-related disability as a result of environmental circumstances rather than personal weaknesses. It is imperative that this phenomenon be understood in the scope of how it plays out in social institutions. Investigating this phenomenon and what it means in educational institutions is therefore important from an academic and practical perspective.

Although the focus of my research is analytical, its application is practical in that it draws on the personal experiences of students and aims to unveil the challenges that are particular to academic accommodation policy and whether it is equitable in relation to Black disabled students. It addresses the phenomenon of marginality in relation to the bureaucratic policies and practices that contribute to the discrimination against Black disabled university students. The research defines a remarkable convergence of representations of Blackness and disability, the internalization of both stigma and anti-Black racism, and at the same time, a mode of resistance to these types of oppression. People at the intersection of Blackness and disability have a long history of being marginalized. My research identifies how their marginalization works in the higher education setting in Canada. It also indicates how this marginality has been normalized in and by Canadian university bureaucracies and how formal documentation is used to support this orientation. Black disabled university students occupy a status of normalized marginality.

The taken-for-granted meanings of Blackness and disability shape educational environments and help to produce, reproduce, and legitimize conceptions of successful and unsuccessful students. The Black disabled individual is seen as being highly dependent on the government and having a lack of economic options. Black university students with disabilities do not necessarily experience their status as central to their selves. However, it has implications for their life. This research has discussed how policies are developed that affect the accommodation of Black disabled students and pointed to the many challenges Black students with disabilities face in the university environment. Black students with disabilities face many of these challenges because of bureaucratic procedures surrounding academic accommodations in higher education. Their marginalization has been embedded in the practices of the institution. Analysis of the experiences of students in my research exposes the ways the university as an institution reinforces their marginalization. The discrimination they experienced is similar to the discrimination faced by Black and disabled scholars elsewhere, both historically and in the present moment. This is evidence that discrimination has several layers. Just as people themselves can be discriminatory and act in ways that marginalize individuals, practices of institutions can have a similar effect; people acting as agents of the institutions in professional roles may not even notice that they are perpetuating the discrimination that is embedded in the systems they work within. The Black disabled students who experience marginalization and discrimination often perceive themselves as needing to become invisible to assume their rightful place. Overall, my research indicates that more must be done to meet the needs of the Black disabled students in institutional settings. The protection of rights in these institutions is such that it is too easy for them to be violated structurally. There is a paternalistic element inherent in several of the social structures we work and learn within. To achieve true equality, it is important that people work together to transcend these structural barriers so there can be a transformation of the ways institutions work.

As previously discussed, my personal experience with the accommodation evaluation and screening process with the Accessibility Services office aligns with those of several of the students. Students differ immensely in many respects. However, the disabled students' differences are given a label and stigmatized as a departure from normalcy. Marginalized students have assumed agency and distanced themselves from stigmatized status by using their developing identities for strategic purposes (Douglas et al., 2021; Loutzenheiser & Erevelles, 2019; Williams, 2008, p. 93). I commiserate with the student who defiantly stated, "I ain't disabled." Our collective disabilities do not define us as human beings. We are individuals; we are all "I's."

In my own case, I see that my personal struggles with the colonial mindset and continued anti-Black racism overshadow the labels placed on me because of my Blackness. My personal resistance to these, though not inconsequential, is only a minor part of the resistance that I and the students in this research must continue to enact. We are navigating a university institution that feels the incessant need to label, categorize, and control a population of the student body.

The continued marginalization of Black students with disabilities remains embedded in the education system. Black disabled students are marginalized by faculty and administration. The nature of this marginalization creates a learning environment where the student perceives mentors as not trusting them and where requests for accommodations are viewed suspiciously by staff. The design of the system makes it difficult to access accommodations, which makes the performance of Black and/or disabled students more difficult. However, as Titchkosky (2011) asserts, "We can wonder about what is really meant when people talk about access, struggle for inclusion, or even get surprised when issues of access arise" (p. 9). The learning environment is a threatening space rather than a safe space. Students feel as though being Black or disabled makes them a target for discrimination by their professors and the administrators whose duty it is to facilitate access to resources that the non-disabled and non-Black either do not require or have readily available.

My research uncovered that Black disabled students at the university often hide or do not mention their disabilities to avoid stigmatization by professors and administration. Black students with disabilities in the university system often see their opportunities as coming with significant barriers. These barriers are microaggressions that make the learning environment hostile (Levchak, 2018; Morales, 2021; Pierce, 1970; Solórzano et al., 2000). One of the 12 interviewees noted that while the university boasts that it is diverse, anti-Black racism has become normalized to the point that peers, administrators, and faculty do not see the abuse (Sarah). My own experience with faculty has led me to similar beliefs.

Not only is the marginalization of Black disabled students perpetuated by the education system, but it is also embedded in its function. My research shows that the operations of marginalization and discrimination in the educational institution are not simply "accidents" of social interaction but are processes that serve the interests of powerful institutions. The education system is designed in such a way that faculty are expected to monitor and assess student performance individually and as a group. One way this is achieved is through inquiry in the classroom. One of the participants experienced classroom microaggressions when their professor referred to some students as "smart monkeys." This was a dehumanizing comment for some students in the class who have experienced being referred to as animals because of their race. The lack of sensitivity of faculty to this issue is a microaggression because it recalls old racist traits even if it is intended to be a positive observation on performance. For Black disabled students, this can impact their perceptions of the educational institution because it contributes to the idea that certain categories of students are not really people. This microaggression can also lead the student to draw implications about whether they are a "smart monkey" or a "not-smart monkey," which for the student, would be an even more challenging suggestion of inferiority and marginality.

Because the marginalization and discrimination of Black students has become an established feature of the education system, it is a complex issue. There are no simple solutions for the problems caused by the marginalization, which is, in turn, caused by the structure and processes embedded in this education system. However, it is important to recognize that the problem exists and to begin to theorize how it could be confronted and dismantled. There is no panacea for the problems created by this marginalization and discrimination; however, it is important to begin now by exploring what potential solutions exist and how these solutions could be implemented. In my own experience, the classroom is one area to address and the administration of university policy and procedure is another. Barriers created by a lack of accommodation can be reinforced by the ways the policy may be manipulated by administration to make the work of students increasingly difficult.

My personal experiences with being a Black person with a disability in the university setting were similar to those of the participants in this research. However, I feel that a discussion of my own experiences can shed further light on the feelings that Black and disabled students have when participating in the university system. The university system is structured to act both with ableism and anti-Black racism. The students in my research discerned instances of systemic racism and ableism and its manifestation in the behavior of agents of the system. Holistically, the system follows a colonial path in which racist and ableist views are accepted, and there is still an absence of mechanisms present in it to protect those who are its victims. The microaggressions that I experienced in the university setting were significant in nature. A reflective discussion of those experiences and others like them within the discussion of the challenges that students face in academia can facilitate a greater understanding of the difficulties that Black disabled people experience when they seek an academic career. My research reveals that the University of Toronto is failing Black disabled students through its academic accommodation policies and practices. It also indicates that the marginalization of Black disabled students is normalized through the routine orders of accommodation processes. Ultimately, this research shows how categories of "Blackness" and "disability" circumscribe educational opportunities for students so labeled. These categories are typically informed by anti-Blackness and biomedical versions of disability that frame it as an "individual lack," which conceals the complex ways hierarchies of power are enabled by the social construction of normalcy. The research discusses how the impact of colonialism and structural inequities within the social placement of Blackness and disability continue to produce injustice in university settings.

The Problem of Bureaucracy

A key issue is that while spokespeople for the bureaucracy regularly espouse beliefs associated with the elimination of marginalization, that marginalization continues to be the consequence of the various ways the university pursues "inclusion" and can be described as a systemic barrier to students' academic achievement. The system is in a spot where marginalization is acknowledged as a problem, yet, students are oftentimes expected to negotiate these accommodations with their professors. Accommodation for disabled students persists as a problem because it is easier for people in the bureaucracy to *say* they own up to the problems than it is to actually address them. The question arises: Why are students' classroom experiences disconnected from the academic accommodation process? As Titchkosky (2011) reminds us, "When disability is taken as something that basically does not belong, it allows for the management of disability as an exception" (p. 34) and "[where] the assertions of inclusion help to normalize conceptions of those who are *essentially excludable*" (p. 39). While some systemic changes do happen, they are typically conservative and fail to address the fundamental factors affecting the issue of marginalization. This research describes what several of these problems are and how they have impacted Black disabled students who have been marginalized by the design of the university system. It is not enough to take ownership of a problem; leadership must be taken by people in the system in order for the systems of accommodation to be transformed.

In this book, I have described the problem of systemic marginalization and how it is that the actors in the system deal with and speak about changes; but the problems persist in spite of their actions. The changes attempted are insufficient and ineffective. The qualitative investigation was designed to explain the inadequacy that persists in the accommodations available to Black disabled individuals and the failures of this university to adequately address them. The ways that students and members of the bureaucracy interact were explored to probe the meaning of being Black and disabled in a university system where accommodation is understood to be necessary for these students. The issues of policy and the way it sustains the university, as well as the marginalization of Black disabled students despite efforts to do otherwise, are key elements of this book.

From a practical standpoint, the objective of this research is to inspire reflection among people in the university system so that we can consider how its bureaucracy has reinforced marginalization of Black disabled students and determine ways to correct the matter. To do this, I proposed some ideas about why the problem exists and suggested the foundation of a framework for considering the problem. By approaching this problem through the scope of deep, immersive discussion with marginalized people in the university and a review of the documentation that supports university standards and practices, I give the reader a foundation for understanding how this problem plays out in practice. While this research describes the problem of marginalization in relation to a case of the bureaucracy of one particular university, the problem is one that permeates North American culture and can be observed in other institutions, even those beyond the university system. For this reason, this book contributes to understanding how intersectional marginalization happens in different places in society.

In this book, I have shown that a strong sense of conflict arises between Black disabled students at the University of Toronto and the university's accommodation system. For example, the people in the university do appear to care about marginalized students, yet there is insufficient thought about what disabled students experience and how the impact of colonialism continues to inform this experience. Nor does the university consider the social construction of *normal* ways of being a student. The problem is one of the values and methods being so deeply ingrained and unexamined in the system that there needs to be some aggressive reflection and intervention for there to be change. The bureaucracy wants to maintain itself, and the changes that are necessary to deal with the issue of marginalization would require actors in the system to reject complacency. Neither the Black disabled student nor the bureaucrats who deal with them yet understand why conditions cannot be improved. To defend the academic accommodation policies for students with disabilities in this university, the bureaucrats say, "We *have* done more, and the problem is solved." On the other hand, noticing how, current forms of assistance are a problem maker requires students to understand the aims and interests of the overall system—a system steeped in hierarchies of power and generated by bureaucratic needs to classify, survey, and control.

Here, I have articulated an understanding of why that is and considered the implications of this situation, particularly at the University of Toronto. Students must understand that universities can do more for them, but this improved treatment for disabled students must first be valued. The problem is that the university is focused on its economic value rather than its value to the students. Change is necessary for all parts of the bureaucracy to be satisfied, including students and members of the system. Overall, the changes that must be undertaken have to happen at the core. This will take people engaging the system and transforming it to regard the needs of these disabled students as simply a different starting point for their studies in an institution that has many such starting points. While this prospect is daunting, without transformative change, the "solutions" will continue to produce little more than problems and perpetuate unresolved issues. Black disabled students will not have access to the educational institution in ways that adequately support their ability to become successful students.

References

Arday, J. (2018). Dismantling power and privilege through reflexivity: Negotiating normative Whiteness, the Eurocentric curriculum and racial micro-aggressions within the Academy. *Whiteness and Education, 3*(2), 141–161. Retrieved from https://doi.org/10.1080/23793406.2019.1574211.

Bratman, E., & DeLince, W. (2022). Dismantling white supremacy in environmental studies and sciences: An argument for anti-racist and decolonizing pedagogies. *Journal of Environmental Studies and Sciences, 12*. Available at: https://doi.org/10.1007/s13412-021-00739-5.

Chordiya, R., & Protonentis, A. (2024). Healing from intersectional white supremacy culture and ableism: Disability justice as an antidote. *Journal of Social Equity and Public Administration, 2*(1), 127–152. https://doi.org/10.24926/jsepa.v2i1.4856.

Connor, D., Ferri, B., & Annamma, S. (2016). *DisCrit: Disability studies and critical race theory in education.* Teachers College Press.

Curtiz, M. (Director). (1942). *Casablanca* [Film]. Warner Bros. Pictures.

Douglas, D. (2022). At the crossroads, Black disabled lives do matter: Intersections of race and disability in special education. *Johns Hopkins University, 3*(1).

Douglas, P., Runswick-Cole, K., Ryan, S., & Fogg, P. (2021). Mad mothering: Learning from the intersections of madness, mothering, and disability. *Journal of Literary & Cultural Disability Studies, 15*(1), 39–56.

Foucault, M. (1995). *Discipline and punish: The birth of the prison.* Trans. Alan Sheridan. Random House.

George, R. C., Maier, R., & Robson, K. (2020). Ignoring race: A comparative analysis of education policy in British Columbia and Ontario. *Race Ethnicity and Education, 23*(2), 159–179.

Hanisch, C. (2006). *The personal is political: The women's liberation movement classic with a new explanatory introduction.* http://webhome.cs.uvic.ca/~mserra/AttachedFiles/PersonalPolitical.pdf

Harris, J. (2021, July 26). *Reckoning with race and disability.* SSRN. https://papers.ssrn.com/sol3/papers.cfm?abstract_id=3878540.

Joyce, S. J. A., & Abdou, E. D. (2023). Dismantling curricular statues: Critically examining Anti-Black racism in representations of Ancient Africa in Canadian textbooks. *Canadian Journal of Education/Revue canadienne de l'éducation, 46*(4), 1051–1082. Retrieved from: https://doi.org/10.53967/cje-rce.5793.

Levchak, C. C. (2018). Microaggressions, macroaggressions, and modern racism in higher education. In *Microaggressions and modern racism* (pp. 85–104). Palgrave Macmillan.

Loutzenheiser, L. W., & Erevelles, N. (2019). "What's disability got to do with it?": Crippin' educational studies at the intersections. *Educational Studies, 55*(4), 375–386.

Morales, E. (2021). "Beasting" at the battleground: Black students responding to racial microaggressions in higher education. *Journal of Diversity in Higher Education, 14*(1), 72.

Morgan, J. (2023). On the relationship between race and disability. *Harv. CR-CLL Rev., 58*, 663. Retrieved from https://journals.law.harvard.edu/crcl/wp-content/uploads/sites/80/2023/09/HLC202_Morgan.pdf.

Pickens, T. (2013). "It's a Jungle Out There:" Blackness and disability in Monk. *Disability Studies Quarterly, 33*(3). Retrieved from https://dsq-sds.org/index.php/dsq/article/view/3391/3269.

Pierce, C. (1970). Offensive mechanisms: The vehicle for microaggressions. In F. Barbour (Ed.), *The Black seventies* (pp. 265–282). Porter Sargent.

Pieterse, A. L., Lewis, J. A., & Miller, M. J. (2023). Dismantling and eradicating anti-Blackness and systemic racism. *Journal of Counseling Psychology, 70*(3), 235–243. Available at: https://doi.org/10.1037/cou0000660.

Schalk, S. (2022). *Black disability politics*. Duke University Press.

Solórzano, D., Ceja, M., & Yosso, T. (2000). Critical race theory, racial microaggressions, and campus racial climate: The experiences of African American college students. *Journal of Negro Education, 69*(1–2), 60–73.

Titchkosky, T. (2000). Disability studies: The old and the new. *Canadian Journal of Sociology, 25*(2), 197–224.

Titchkosky, T. (2011). *The question of access: Disability, space, meaning*. University of Toronto Press.

Williams, R. (2008). The cultural contexts of collective action: Constraints, opportunities and the symbolic life of social movements. In D. Snow, Sarah A. Soule, & Hanspeter Kriesi (Eds.), *The Blackwell companion to social movements* (pp. 91–115). Blackwell-John Wiley & Sons.

Chapter 7

Future Directions

The objective of the research discussed in this book was to contribute an evidence-based guide to understanding what it means to be Black and disabled in higher education. It incorporates empirical research with personal narratives as a way to develop a robust understanding of the problem. Research that is focused on the intersectionality of Blackness and disability in higher education is sorely limited, and the work of respected scholars in Black and disability studies that is available indicates that racialized people have differential experiences in education, particularly in higher education. Instead, this book focuses on how Blackness and disability are connected through power relations in education and associated social institutions. It draws on scholarly work spanning several decades, highlighting existing theoretical models and concepts of Black identity. This book employs a disruptive framework aimed against oppressive hegemonic discourses in education and pedagogic practice. An important element of this research was to understand the distinct intersectional experiences of Black disabled students in several different contexts to determine whether social forces are impacting these students, and if so, to determine common themes in their experience of them.

Looking forward to the future, research into equity and inclusion for Black students with disabilities needs to consider how both intentional and structural anti-Blackness impacts mental health, disability, and student welfare policy in higher education. A review of the limited literature associated with Black disabled students provides evidence that higher education is especially problematic for students with subject position categories at the intersection of Blackness and disability. The literature is largely silent on accommodation politics and practices for the disabled and/or how they impact Black students. This absence of published materials on Blackness and disability stems from scholarly inattention due to a long tradition of the institution as a white, able, largely male elite.

The educational system is plagued by anti-Blackness and ableism, as suggested by many of the research participants, and this continues to be a central problem. A significant body of the scholarly literature illustrates that educational institutions preserve and perpetuate a system of structured inequities based on Blackness, disability, or gender (Collins, 2015; McKittrick, 2015; Schalk, 2022; Titchkosky & Michalko, 2009). Elements of the education setting still place a value on being both an able-bodied and non-racialized individual. Thus, the university system carries vestiges of what education was designed to accomplish in the scope of preparing for economic success and the people the system was designed to accommodate. Barriers persist for Black disabled students who must struggle to overcome to obtain a place in an education program and to succeed in it. At both the secondary and postsecondary levels, there is still institutional resistance to approaches to access that promote full inclusion and equity. Education is, of course, critical to not only personal and intellectual growth and development but also to attaining economic self-sufficiency.

My hope in this book is that it produces a greater knowledge of the intersection of Blackness and disability and effective conceptual models to understand it, helping others to appreciate the issues of access and accommodation in new ways. Thinking in this way needs to become part of our first instinct, to think critically and interrogate "ableist" or "anti-Black racism" discourses wherever they occur, no matter how subtly they may be represented. We will think more clearly about the situation Black disabled people find themselves in, and about their needs, and incorporate their experiences to deepen our understanding of the operations of political and institutional social forces in shaping the world around us.

Blackness and Disability as the Problem of Identity

The collective experience of the individuals that participated in this investigation addresses the primary deficiencies in policy and the practical application of policy when striving to ensure equality for all university students. The inequities experienced reflect a larger societal problem that has a commonality for all Black students in a postcolonial paradigm, and this is exacerbated when intersected with disability. This research seeks to record and qualitatively examine the experiences of Black university students with disabilities at the University of Toronto and to raise awareness of the inequities that exist due to social conditions of historical origin that continue to influence the students' experiences. The understanding of their individual experiences and their collective understanding of Blackness and disability through the labeling built into the process of meting out the requisite accommodations guaranteed by policy and law is a necessary step toward redress.

The primary goal of society when it comes to disability is prevention, cure, or finally, if the previous two are impossible, to make the individual look and feel as "normal" as possible (Titchkosky & Michalko, 2009, p. 3). Even the Canadian government does not recognize disability as a way of life but as an "abnormal" condition (Titchkosky & Michalko, 2009, p. 5). In this way, it places disability in a different category than other groups it considers disadvantaged due to other life circumstances. Taylor (2011) draws interesting parallels between how animals and disabled people are treated in showing how some bodies (human or animal) are treated as normal, some as broken or dysfunctional, and some as food. She finds that disabled people are often compared to animals in metaphorical terms when describing their disability and the differences between their bodies and those of "normal" people. However, these paradigms of normalcy and exclusion have not been left unchallenged. Smith (2000) relates how perceptions of Black people as criminals and inferior were purposely challenged at the turn of the twentieth century.

For example, thinking about the intersection of Blackness and disability has led to questioning the concept of "normalcy" from which disability, and to an extent Blackness, differs. In the literature, this idea has been roundly criticized, and yet prior research has shown that it is often still used on a practical level when disabled students are treated as less able rather than as living with another form of human experience for whom education requires reasonable accommodations (Harpur & Stein, 2018; Liachowitz, 2010; Prema & Dhand, 2019). This is true, particularly for students from populations that have historically been racially marginalized, such as Black Canadians and Indigenous Peoples (Connauton, 2020; McKenzie et al., 2023; Wotherspoon, 2014). The acceptance of these stereotypes, and the creation of commonly accepted terms that are truly nothing more than subtle terms to describe individuals with certain characteristics, are ways that marginalization becomes normalized. For Black disabled students in a university setting, it can be extremely difficult to feel truly accepted and to conform to societal standards. There has been a critical momentum in trying to reconfigure the "intersections" of Blackness and disability (Annamma et al., 2013; Baker, 2019). The attempt to create a dual theory of Blackness and disability has been intriguing since there has been an admitted impasse on these grounds (Annamma et al., 2013). For example, in sociological terms, Black students are three times as likely to be labeled as "mentally retarded" and one and half times more likely to be called "learning disabled" than their white peers (Annamma et al., 2013; Mercer, 2022; Romney, 2019). This is disconcerting and reminds us that the old tenets of racist assumptions are still operative within the medical discourses that determine who is disabled and who is not. There are obvious political and social, let alone moral, grounds on which to challenge these assumptions, and critical reinjection of Black identity theory appears to be more pressing than ever in the field of education. The problem is perhaps not that academics are unaware of theories of racial identity; rather, they have perhaps not always taken into account how medical institutions and authorities have operated under this notion of normativity as a condition of whiteness. This is particularly alarming issue for special education professionals, who need to be made more aware of the "markers of identity" that come into play when discourses of disability are created outside of the academic realm (Annamma et al., 2013, p. 3).

In this regard, I hold a more intersectional approach to disability studies and Black studies, such that I am mindful of how social categories are constructed by specific institutions and discourses (Annamma et al., 2013). In this, I am aligned with theorists who have noted how difficult it is to get beyond the mere "anticategorical" view that sees Blackness as only a social fiction (Annamma et al., 2013, p. 4). This seems inadequate for addressing how the educational system has labeled or restricted people based upon Blackness, and this is true also of so-called disabled students. My concern is with how Black disabled students may exist between categories and, as a result, may be subjected to a different discourse of ableism, one that is informed by racist or bigoted assumptions (Annamma et al., 2013). That there appears to be a "perpetual over-representation of how Black students within dis/ability categories" (Annamma et al., 2013, p. 22) is a serious concern for professionals and practitioners in the field of education.

This is a sociological problem, but I would argue that by retheorizing identity in the field of Black studies, we may be able to reach a better understanding of how Black disabled students are seen through these various gazes and how they conceive of themselves within these institutions. Hall's (2000) question of "Who needs identity?" is pertinent here. I agree with him that we do not need to get rid of the adjectives Black or disabled; rather, we need to reconceptualize identity as a relationship "between subjects and discursive practices" (p. 16). That is, Black identity can be better theorized in education by placing it in what I earlier called a dialectic of gazes that are informed by the practical and theoretical language we use to describe conditions or experiences (Oliver, 1996). This view of Black identity fits in, I argue, with both identity-based approaches and post-modern ideas of performing or enacting identity.

This means that I agree that social disability is a fluid state and also a fluid subject of academic criticism (Barnartt, 2010). The fluidity here suggests that racial and disabled identities can intersect and at times remain independent of one another, meaning that one can reclaim a racial identity that is not necessarily dependent upon being a disabled person (Barnartt, 2010). This is an important point because it opens up a space to discuss disability as a changing term depending upon context. This view certainly admits that the notion of identity remains elusive, but it also admits that certain identities can be reclaimed as the discourses surrounding them alter (Bauman, 2004). It recognizes that one must look for the "fissures" in the "totalizing view" of those markers, which have historically come to define Black people's experience as a transmitted product of European culture (Samuels, 2014, p. 7). Samuels' (2014) analysis is helpful in showing how a concept of fluidity speaks against this embedded notion that "personhood is biological," and one can understand how remnants of this nineteenth century view are operative in many of the discourses surrounding identity of the self (p. 7).

This is indeed dangerous ground for marking the disabled body or the racialized body because the presumption is that there is some way to detect these identities as one might view a fingerprint (Samuels, 2014). The political implications in assuming a biological or physiological definition of Blackness and disability are obvious to critics perhaps, but there is often an uncritical acceptance of some of these ideas in the discourse of disability (Samuels, 2014).

Sandahl (2004) reconceptualizes Black identity as something that is not just performed but also constituted by relations with others and the body politic. She speaks of a potential resistance along these lines by talking about "dismodernism" as a development of the civil rights disability movement (p. 581). This view is in accord with what I am arguing here because it acknowledges the fluidity of identity, but it also notes that what we have in common is our differences, which can lead to transforming the self (Sandahl, 2004).

Sandhal's (2004) analysis in conjunction with Butler's (1993) notion of performativity is operative for my view of the intersections of Black and disability identities because it leads to an awareness of how the body is watched and cared for in spaces and in discourse. In exploring the idea of the dismodern ethic, Sandhal (2004) argues "for a commonality of bodies within the notion of difference" and thus for caring about the processes of embodiment as a central concern (p. 581).

Nonetheless, the stratification of Canadian society, along the lines of disability, Blackness, and class remains a pressing issue, and this structure is reproduced in educational institutions. These educational systems are reflecting the anti-Black racism that remains in the larger society. This is a problem because it is a systemic denial of what it means to be Black and has resulted in the elimination of an understanding of the phenomenon of Blackness. Only by opening up the discussion of Blackness to these other interpretative categories of social oppression and injustice can we achieve institutional change. Black identity is a contentious social and political construct; it is important to understand how both oppressors and the resisting forces advocating social and political justice conceptualize the Black identity in relation to the physical body. The relationship between a global education system that reinforces colonial and corporate power upon a colonized Black body and the Canadian education system that constructs normalcy as able-bodied and imposes this value system as normative upon students with disabilities allows us to understand the profound and negative impact of this value system upon students. I suggest that this impact goes far beyond stigmatizing or labeling students. Along with other disability scholars, we witness the construction of normalcy in the classroom—with able-bodies as normative—and how it can result in an entire cohort of Black disabled students seeing their "human capital" as being of secondary worth (Davis, 2002; Rizvi, 2009; Wotherspoon, 2014). The long-term damage of this system to Canadian society can be inferred, again by analogy, when we consider the worldwide effect of the damage done by colonialism and unchecked corporate hegemony.

Behind my work here is the assumed existence of a hegemonic educational system in Toronto and of globally exported constructs of Blackness and disabilities as problems in need of a solution; indeed, "for which solutions *must* be sought" (Titchkosky & Michalko, 2009, p. 2). Of course, while the historical record shows that the education systems in Western countries have tended to serve the interests of class and cultural elites, many educators do not want "disability" to be anything and in fact recognize it as a phenomenon of social exclusion. It is truly remarkable that marginalized and oppressed Black disabled students can be held solely responsible for their own marginalization and social exclusion. Thus, the marginalized learn their "place" in education; but most importantly, they learn that they may never be equal. Indeed, the only hope they are given of even approaching acceptance is to disavow and destroy their own selves and seek equality. What is clear is that education is used in many forms to normalize racial oppression and, like law, to set in place a plantation colonial system that asserts and reaffirms the inherent superiority of the oppressor (McKittrick, 2015 Walcott, 2021). Evidence in my research suggests that students at the intersection of Blackness and disability face problems and barriers in the university environment that students at other intersections will never face. In this context, in order "to implement social change that embraces" inclusion and equity in the university system, we should begin by learning from the experiences of marginalized students who occupy multiple disadvantaged positions within educational institutions (Titchkosky, 2011, p. 12).

Seeing how disability and Blackness are culturally constructed allows us to also explore how normalcy is similarly culturally constructed—and yet obscured—as a taken-for-granted foundation for social, economic, and cultural privilege in our society. Critical Black studies and disability studies are effective as an equity resource in university systems based on power and inequity because they illustrate methods to challenge ableism, racial discrimination, and oppression (Erevelles, 2019; Schalk, 2022). These are normalized and deeply embedded in university policies, practices, and patterns. However, how they are experienced by Black disabled students has given these students a "unique kind of burden which is both 'symbolic' and 'material,' derived from the notion of ... Blackness or [disability] as a cultural trope and a set of subject positions" (Mapedzahama & Kwansah-Aidoo, 2017, p. 5; see also Farrugia, 2010). Critical Black studies theorists suggest that anti-Black racism and institutional discrimination in Canadian society is a complex and insidious phenomenon that cannot be easily combated. This is especially so given the Canadian state's denial of its existence.

Thus, the fact that racism has clear economic "benefits" for the capitalist corporate elite of our society is all the more troubling. Given the deep roots of racism and racist exclusion in our culture, together with the "usefulness" of the practice of excluding vulnerable Black students from full participation in university environments, the challenges of taking action against racism and ableism in our society are arguably as great as they ever were in the past—they are merely different, in complex ways. This analysis allows us to understand not only how people talk about Blackness in our culture, but how this talk, this policy, and these practices are deeply implicated in its power dynamics and, in particular, in structures of domination based on coloniality, disability, and normalcy. The problem of the accommodation and marginalization of Black disabled students is not only perpetuated by the university system but is also part of how it functions normally. Accommodation can be understood as a systemic process of marginalization.

Accommodation is power that administrators hold over students' heads to establish control and illustrates that systemic marginality is a default position for Black disabled students. Providing accommodation is a form of power operating through the normative orders of university bureaucratic processes. In Titchkosky's (2011) words, power is used as a "justification to perform acts of discrimination and exclusion" (p. 86). This power is used as a way to marginalize these students, particularly in the scope of their bodies. My aim is to raise a collective awareness of anti-Blackness in negotiating equity in educational opportunities for students with disabilities.

Recommendations

For educational institutions seeking broader cultural change and socially just pedagogies, the classroom represents a critical avenue to long-term success. As I have argued throughout this book, thinking deeply about and challenging categorizations of Blackness and disability and the abled is essential if we are to change the discourse surrounding accommodation access, equity, inclusion, marginality, and pedagogical action in the university system.

We must open up the discussion about Blackness and disability in higher education, as well as other forms of social oppression and injustice, as a necessary step to making higher education more just. To implement change that fully embraces inclusion, diversity, and social justice in its activities, the university needs to learn from the experiences of Black and disabled students. This research aims to give Black students with disabilities a voice to speak about their university experiences. One of the main problems for students with disabilities is the difficulty they experience in accessing the bureaucratic ordering of accommodation through Accessibility Services. One of the problems with how academic accommodations are administered is the lack of accountability and transparency in how students are accommodated. There is also no accountability from the university administration for the ongoing harm caused by anti-Blackness and anti-racism.

A majority of the students who participated in this research expressed their desire to see a more diverse group of Black service providers in the university environment. That is one important recommendation, based on the Black students' personal experiences, but there are many other ways to improve access and equity in services.

Recommendations for Improved University Practices

- Diversify the University of Toronto administration team.
- Develop and implement culturally inclusive education policy initiatives in the curriculum, such as using assistive technology, cultural sensitivity training, Black inclusion, anti-oppression, and social justice.
- Develop and implement processes that include the participation of Black, disabled, and Indigenous voices in decision-making, planning, implementation, evaluation of education programs, services, and equity initiatives.
- Initiate race-based data, strengths and needs assessment data, and anti-Black racism outcome data to inform planning, implementation, and evaluation of all equity, diversity, and inclusion interventions.

- Integrate an equity accessibility lens into strategic planning to ensure anti-Blackness and anti-racism efforts are at the forefront of the university culture.
- Establish an effective oversight committee to ensure that policies, procedures, and communications are consistent with the fundamental principles and practices of equity, anti-racism, diversity, inclusion, and accessibility.
- Administrators and policymakers must encourage cultural diversity, which can help students cultivate a sense of belonging and foster an equitable and accessible learning environment for all future students.

It is important for many institutions that discrimination is addressed in employee agreements, contracts, and regulations that lay out what is expected from employees. For the University of Toronto faculty (2016), Article 9 of their Memorandum of Agreement addresses the issue of discrimination against employees on the bases of several identity categories. These terms cover several layers of identity and are an explicit expression on the part of university administration and executives of protection against unequal treatment for workers on the basis of characteristics that do not undermine their ability to perform work duties.

The point of academic accommodation practices is to address the issue of social disadvantage to work toward greater equality of results. There are both individual and structural reasons for social inequalities, and because of this multitude of reasons, many people are impacted (Chataika, 2018; Wotherspoon, 2014). It would be difficult, if not impossible, to successfully address all these inequalities. For this reason, general policy is designed as a means by which the special needs of students can be addressed generally. It is important that the procession of fair educational opportunity become central because education is considered the key to social and economic rewards and opportunities in society. Equality of access and treatment of students are two key factors that precipitate the equality of rewards and the ability of administrators to move toward socially responsible activities. Wotherspoon (2014) notes that compulsory education is one of the primary ways that the government is able to facilitate the reduction in inequality in Canada because education is a key way for the poor, Indigenous, and disabled to gain access to social and economic opportunities they would not otherwise have access to.

Ultimately, these recommendations aim to reduce anti-Black racism and inequities in higher education institutions. By clearly identifying this problem and how it functions, this research substantively contributes to the body of knowledge on Blackness and disability in higher education and the implication of this for pedagogy and service provision in educational institutions in Canada.

References

Annamma, S. A., Connor, D., & Ferri, B. (2013). Dis/ability critical race studies (DisCrit): Theorizing at the intersections of race and dis/ability. *Race Ethnicity and Education, 16*(1), 1–31.

Baker, L. A. (2019). *Normalizing marginality: A critical analysis of blackness and disability in higher education* [Unpublished doctoral dissertation]. University of Toronto.

Barnartt, S. (Ed.). (2010). *Disability as a fluid state*. Emerald Group Publishing.

Bauman, Z. (2004). *Identity: Conversations with Benedetto Vecchi*. Polity Press.

Butler, J. (1993). *Bodies that matter: On the discursive limits of 'sex'*. New York: Routledge.

Chataika, T. (Ed.). (2018). *The Routledge handbook of disability in Southern Africa*. Routledge.

Collins, P. H. (2015). Intersectionality's definitional dilemmas. *Annual Review of Sociology, 41*, 1–20. https://journals-scholarsportal-info.myaccess.library.utoronto.ca/pdf/03600572/v41inone/1_idd.xml.

Connauton, J. J. (2020). *"It feels like a battle to tell myself that I am worthy of being here": Understanding the racially marginalized student experience in Canadian higher education* [Master's thesis, University of Edmonton]. Education and Research Archive. Retrieved from https://era.library.ualberta.ca/items/5e7c8ee4-4563-407c-9882-fee271c86ae0.

Davis, L. J. (2002). *Bending over backwards: Essays on disability and the body* (Vol. 6). New York University Press.

Erevelles, N. (2019). "Scenes of subjection" in public education: Thinking intersectionally as if disability matters. *Educational Studies, 55*(6), 592–605.

Farrugia, D. (2010). The symbolic burden of homelessness: Towards a theory of youth homelessness as embodied subjectivity. *Journal of Sociology, 47*, 71–87.

Hall, S. (2000). Who needs identity? In P. du Gay, J. Evans, & P. Redman (Eds.), *Identity: A reader* (pp. 15–30). Sage Publications.

Harpur, P., & Stein, M. A. (2018). Universities as disability rights change agents. *NEULJ, 10*, 542.

Liachowitz, C. H. (2010). *Disability as a social construct: Legislative roots*. University of Pennsylvania Press.

Mapedzahama, V., & Kwansah-Aidoo, K. (2017). Blackness as burden? The lived experience of black Africans in Australia. *Sage Open, 7*(3). http://journals.sagepub.com/doi/pdf/10.1177/2158244017720483.

McKittrick, K. (Ed.). (2015). *Sylvia Wynter: On being human as praxis*. Duke University Press.

McKenzie, B., Joseph, J., & Razack, S. (2023). Whiteness, Canadian university athletic administration, and anti-racism leadership: "A bunch of white haired, white dudes in the back rooms." *Qualitative Research in Sport, Exercise and Health, 2*, 1–16.

Mercer, J. R. (2022). *Labeling the mentally retarded: Clinical and social system perspectives on mental retardation*. University of California Press.

Oliver, M. (1996). *Understanding disability: From theory to practice*. St. Martin's Press.

Prema, D., & Dhand, R. (2019). Inclusion and accessibility in STEM education: Navigating the duty to accommodate and disability rights. *Canadian Journal of Disability Studies, 8*(3), 121–141.

Rizvi, F. (2009). Postcolonialism and globalization in education. In R. S. Coloma (Ed.), *Postcolonial challenges in education* (pp. 46–54). Peter Lang.

Romney, L. (2019, October 18). A landmark lawsuit aimed to fix special ed for California's black students. It didn't. *KQED News*. Retrieved from https://www.kqed.org/news/11781032/a-landmark-lawsuit-aimed-to-fix-special-ed-for-californias-black-students-it-didnt.

Samuels, E. (2014). *Fantasies of identification: Disability, gender, race*. New York University Press.

Sandahl, C. (2004). Black man, blind man: Disability, identity, politics and performance. *Theatre Journal, 56*(4), 579–602.

Schalk, S. (2022). *Black disability politics*. Duke University Press.

Smith, S. M. (2000). Looking at oneself through the eyes of others: W.E.B. Du Bois' photographs for the 1900 Paris exposition. *African American Review, 34*(4), 581–599.

Taylor, S. (2011). Beasts of burden: Disability studies and animal rights. *Qui Parle: Critical Humanities and Social Sciences, 19*(2), 191–222.

Titchkosky, T., & Michalko, R. (2009). *Rethinking normalcy: A disability studies reader*. Canadian Scholars' Press.

Titchkosky, T. (2011). *The question of access: Disability, space, meaning*. University of Toronto Press.

Walcott, R. (2021). *On property: Policing, prisons, and the call for abolition* (Vol. 2). Biblioasis.

Wotherspoon, T. (2014). *The sociology of education in Canada: Critical perspectives* (4th ed.). Oxford University Press.

Appendix A

Student Interview Questions

Blackness and Disability in Higher Education

1. Please tell me about your experience of being a Black disabled student at the University of Toronto?
2. What has accessing accommodation been like for you?
3. Have you had any accommodation experiences with administrators? If yes, what has this been like?
4. Have you had any accommodation experiences related to professors or TA's? If yes, what has this been like?
5. In your experience, are there any experiences of marginalization in the university that might be related to being a Black disabled student? If yes, can you tell me a bit more about this?
6. In your perception, what factors do you think have shaped your university experiences?

7. Do you experience Blackness and disability playing out at the University of Toronto in any other ways, or ways you haven't mentioned yet?

Appendix B

List of the Research Participants

	Pseudonym	Year	Level	Discipline
1	Christine	4th year	Undergraduate	Arts and Sciences
2	Lorna	3rd year	PhD	Humanities and Social Sciences
3	Paige	1st year	Masters	Humanities and Social Sciences
4	Stephanie	3rd year	Undergraduate	Arts and Sciences
5	Zaine	2nd year	Masters	Humanities and Social Sciences
6	Kimberly	2nd year	Masters	Humanities and Social Sciences
7	Folake	2nd year	Masters	Humanities and Social Sciences
8	David	4th year	Undergraduate	Arts and Sciences
9	Barry	1st year	Undergraduate	Arts and Sciences
10	Sarah	2nd year	PhD	Sciences
11	Denise	2nd year	Masters	Humanities and Social Sciences
12	Saga	1st year	Undergraduate	Arts and Sciences

Index

Ability 8, 81, 151, 164, 188
Able-bodiedness 125
Ableism 3, 12, 16–18, 52, 109, 113, 147–148, 181, 203, 215–217, 219, 240–241
Ableist 93, 111, 125, 148, 150–151, 156–157, 186, 198, 227, 234
Abnormal 71, 116, 137–138, 151, 210, 235
Abnormality 121
Academic accommodations 2, 4, 17, 94, 146, 163, 175–176, 189, 191, 224, 242
Acceptable 137, 151, 178
Access 20
Accessibility 138, 145, 166
Accessibility Services Office 12, 17, 64, 93, 141, 163–164, 170–176, 178, 183, 190–191, 201–209, 225
Accountability 242
Adjustments 166
Administration 1, 15–16, 138, 144, 148, 152, 170, 208, 221, 226–227, 242–243
Amputate 205

Anti-Blackness 1, 14, 16, 37–39, 149–151, 215–218, 228, 234, 241–243
Anti-Black racism 1–3, 9, 22, 39, 47, 135, 138, 146–155, 183–184, 215, 218, 224–227, 242, 244
Anticategorical 14, 237
Appeal 2
Appendix A-Student Interview Questions 247
Arbitrary 66, 117, 184
Authoritarian 28

Barriers 1–2, 17, 22, 62, 109, 117, 123, 148–149, 166, 180, 192–193, 203, 225–227, 240
Battlefields 223
Bell curve 137, 139
Belonging 17, 129, 131, 133, 144, 219, 243
Blackness 1–16, 19–22, 33–41, 43, 49, 51–53, 55, 57, 59, 62–63, 65, 122, 126–130, 197–198, 233–244, 247–248

Black students with disabilities 2–3, 5, 9–10, 14–16, 93, 101, 115, 165–166, 174–175, 180–181, 201, 242
Body politic 238
Brokenness 63, 72, 85
Bureaucracy 3–4, 8–9, 15–17, 109, 113, 152, 156–157, 164–166, 228–230
Bureaucratic policies and practices 8, 10–11, 15–17, 19, 22, 113, 224
Bureaucratization 166, 173
Bursary for Students with Disabilities 171

Capitalism 12, 42, 189, 217
Caribbean 49, 53–55, 65
Categories 9–10, 12, 74–77, 79, 90, 202, 222–223, 227–228, 239 243
Classroom 2–3, 17–18, 112, 136–139, 142–144, 163–165, 169–170, 199, 241
Colonialism 3, 11, 40, 43, 45–49, 51–55, 63, 90, 94, 131, 145, 149, 199, 228, 230, 239
Coloniality 28, 48, 181, 241
Color-blindness 144
Complexity 3, 5, 8, 11–16, 52, 54, 56, 58, 60, 62, 64, 232, 234, 236, 238, 240, 242, 244
Compulsory heterosexuality 42
Construction site 134
Cultural capital 136
Cure 64, 70–71, 75–76, 181, 235

Decolonization 43, 45, 52, 55
Definition 68, 98, 169, 208
Deviance 65, 70, 79, 88, 100, 134–135, 137, 196, 199
Diagnosis 18, 65, 70, 76, 78, 102, 168–169, 216, 222
Differential 20, 22, 28, 38–39, 65 233
Disability 1–11, 13–22, 45, 47, 52, 61–79, 81, 83, 133–140, 147, 149, 151–153, 156–157, 230, 233–242, 244, 247–248
Disablement 186

Disadvantage 20, 29, 123, 147, 174, 210, 243
Discipline 18, 52, 98–99, 117, 127, 147, 166, 249
Discrimination 1, 3, 5–6, 10, 13–15, 19–20, 141, 144–145, 147, 150, 183–184, 187, 217–220, 224–227, 240–241, 243
Discriminatory label 64

Disorder 64, 66–69, 91, 121, 221
Diversity 1, 18, 30, 42, 48, 63, 138, 140, 144–145, 218, 242–243
DNA replication 134
Docile body/docile bodies 98–99
Double consciousness 128–129, 131, 148

Economic benefits 136
Education 1, 3–4, 8–11, 34–39, 43–44, 55, 61–62, 148–149, 168–169, 184, 186–188, 224, 239–244, 247
Educational environments 224
Egalitarian 64, 141, 145, 201
Eligibility 8, 22, 112, 169, 173, 175–177, 202, 205, 209
Embodiment 15, 72–74, 120, 130, 138, 203, 239
Enclosure 222
Environmental 74, 218, 223
Epistemological control 9
Equality 18–19, 30, 49, 157, 199, 219, 225, 235, 240, 243
Equilibrium 63
Equity 1, 4–5, 65, 138, 150, 152–153, 166, 178, 191, 219, 222, 234, 240–243
Exceptionalism 18
Exclusion 8, 18, 38, 47–48, 154, 165, 168, 178, 180, 215, 217, 219, 223, 236, 240–241
Exclusionary 189
Expected student 113
Exploitation 46, 53, 111, 167, 173, 201

Figure 1.1 - Blackness and Disability Research Flowchart 21

INDEX

Gatekeeping 174, 217–218
Gifted learners 136

Habit worlds 186
Harassment 149, 151, 153, 186
Hegemonic 46, 77–78, 80, 95–96, 194–195, 203, 210, 219, 233, 239
Hidden 101, 169
Hierarchy 19, 49, 132–133, 149, 155, 167, 173, 205–206, 209, 219, 228, 230
Hypervisibility 29–30, 35

Identity 3, 5–6, 33–35, 37, 40–42, 47, 51, 208, 215, 222–223, 225, 233, 235–239, 243
Impairment 17–18, 63, 67, 70, 72, 117, 120, 122, 124, 133, 168, 172, 186, 208
Impression management 96
Inadequacy 3, 136, 229
Inclusionary 189
Inferiority 35, 39, 43, 45, 47, 62, 81, 90, 100, 114, 134, 149, 180 227
Institutional bureaucratic practices 7–11, 13, 15–17, 19, 22, 113, 126, 155, 165, 170, 177, 181, 192, 224, 241
Institutional ethnography 16
Interlocking 115
Intersectionality 3, 6, 9–10, 12–17, 19, 22, 62, 85–87, 89, 91, 93, 95, 97, 99, 101, 103, 105, 233
Intracategorical 14
Investigation 4, 6, 13–15, 19, 28, 99, 119, 131, 148, 170, 229, 235
Invisible 4–5, 29–31, 42, 72, 93–94

Jamaica 40–45, 48–52, 73, 88–89 112
Judge 101, 143, 190
Judgmental 68

Labeled 65, 68, 90, 99, 101, 121, 123, 140, 222, 228, 236–237
Labeling 20, 28, 37, 65, 77, 99–101, 195, 204–205, 209, 235 239

Language 11, 44–48, 99, 114, 136, 139, 156, 180, 207, 237
Learning assessment 64, 164–165, 183, 201, 204–205
Legitimacy 41, 116, 194
Liberatory contestation 74–75
Lip service 126, 152
Looking-glass self 143

Man enough 62
Marginal 91, 120, 136
Marginality 8, 13, 15, 21, 71, 87, 112, 119, 133, 148, 170, 182, 194–195, 207, 210, 224, 227, 241
Marginalization 3–5, 7, 9, 14–15, 114, 119–120, 210, 216, 221, 223–231, 236, 240–241, 247
Masculinity 40–42, 52, 54, 62–64, 68–69, 73, 85, 88–89, 95
Mass media 118
Master/slave dialectic 131–132
Medical model 17, 70–71, 91, 117, 137, 169, 208
Medication 38, 64–65, 76, 115
Medicine 66, 75, 199
Metaphor 55, 79, 86, 97
Microaggression 2, 29–30, 38, 108, 141–146, 148, 151, 215, 217, 219–220, 226–228
Mind the gap 222
Mission Statement 138
Mono-system analysis 13

Navigate/navigating 91, 225
Normal 64, 72, 79, 87, 90, 93, 114–115, 121, 133–138
Normalcy 4, 7, 15, 22, 66, 68, 75–76, 79, 86, 134–137, 188, 207–210, 219, 225, 228, 236, 239–241
Normality 64–66, 134–135, 137, 181, 209
Normalization 8, 11, 21, 43, 52, 71, 151, 167, 219

Normalizing 74, 100, 119, 167, 189, 203, 210
Normate 135–136, 139
Normative 37, 65, 79, 87, 97, 100, 113, 120, 129, 133–134, 136, 139, 188, 239, 241
Notion of zones, 67

Ontario Student Assistance Program (OSAP) 172–177 192, 209
Overrepresented 28, 168
Over-sensitivity 145

Pass 79–81, 96–98, 171, 205
Passing 80, 91, 96, 98, 140, 153, 196, 198
Paternal abandonment 40
Perform 78, 126
Performance 77–80
Performativity 96–97, 238
Performing 78, 95, 138–139, 141 237
Personal is political 78, 223
Philosophical 28, 131, 207
Physical abuse 48
Pitfalls 130
Plantation logic 167
Plantation mentality 20–21, 149, 166–168, 183, 190–191, 201
Plantation slavery 49
Police 38, 127, 154, 216
Post-colonial 45, 47, 127, 129–130
Postcolonialism 47
Postmodern 129
Post-traumatic stress disorder (PTSD) 64–71, 76, 78, 102, 221–223
Power 127–128, 134, 174, 180, 184, 187
Prejudice 16, 35, 37, 41, 45, 49, 88, 131, 153, 171, 181, 190, 192, 203, 217–218
Privileged 62, 114, 132, 134, 137, 149, 179
Problem people 71, 76, 126, 199, 223
Professors 16, 101, 111–112, 122, 151, 170–172, 187–188, 193, 196, 226, 228, 247
Prove 180
Provisional 14, 76

Psychological 44–45, 54–55, 67, 70, 129, 131–132, 142, 167, 184, 204–205, 216
Punishment 41, 102, 183, 205 209

Qualitative research 229, 235

Racially profiling 154
Racism 1–3, 6, 9, 12, 181, 183–184, 224–227, 235, 239–244
Rastafarian 51
Real and the representational 77–78, 221–223
Recognition 5, 47, 54, 78, 86–87, 100, 132, 143, 194–195, 223
Re-colonizing 74
Rehabilitation 75, 96–97
Religion/christianity 35, 44, 48–51
Research questions 9

Security guard 109, 153
Segregation 65, 94, 101, 198
Self-appointed white authorities 154–155
Self-identification 77, 123, 165 195
Sense of place 20, 183
Shortcoming 164, 166, 183, 199, 201, 203
Single attribute 95, 194
Smart monkey 140, 145, 227
Social actors 194–195
Social justice 6, 112, 242
Social models 87
Social reproduction 117, 189
Standard 66, 137
Stigma 20, 22, 96, 99, 112, 123, 139–140, 165, 192–199, 203–205, 224
Stigmatization 41, 65, 70, 79, 98–99, 192–193, 196–197, 200, 223, 226
Stigmatized 8, 137, 140, 146, 183, 195–196, 200, 225
Stigmatizing 91, 102, 111, 139, 155, 196–198, 204, 239
Subhuman 28, 47, 156
Subjectivity 28–29, 116, 118

Surveillance 116, 150–151, 155, 176, 184–186
Suspicious 76, 116
Symptoms 66–69, 76
Systemic 1–2, 5, 13, 37, 118, 126, 215, 217, 219, 227–229, 239, 241

Table 3.1- list of the research participants 249
Tabula rasa 73
Testing environment 207
Therapy 70, 76
Tragedy/tragedies 63, 75–76 114
Transparency 242
Trauma 8, 19, 65, 69, 149, 206 217

Treatment 38–39, 45, 119, 146, 155, 157, 179, 185, 191, 203, 216, 221, 230, 243

Under repair 5
University system 3, 10, 109, 149, 191, 226–227, 229, 234, 240–241

Visibility 1, 4–5, 101
Visible 4, 27, 29, 94, 193
Visible minorities 4, 187
Vulnerability 2, 119, 122, 185–186, 202
Vulnerable 40, 73, 119, 185–186, 192, 204, 241
The Wizard of Oz 136

www.ingramcontent.com/pod-product-compliance
Lightning Source LLC
Chambersburg PA
CBHW061710300426
44115CB00014B/2624